Preoperative Cardiac Assessment

Edited by
Dennis T. Mangano, PhD, MD

Professor and Vice Chairman
Department of Anesthesia
University of California, San Francisco
San Francisco, California

With 8 contributors

J. B. LIPPINCOTT COMPANY
Philadelphia

Grand Rapids New York St. Louis San Francisco
London Sydney Tokyo

Preoperative Cardiac Assessment

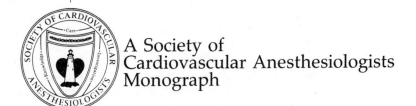

A Society of
Cardiovascular Anesthesiologists
Monograph

Acquisitions Editor: Nancy L. Mullins
Copy Editor: Carol A. Florence
Project Editor: Kathy Crown
Indexer: Victoria Boyle
Art Director: Susan Hess Blaker
Design Coordinator: Ellen C. Dawson
Cover and Interior Designer: Ellen C. Dawson
Production Manager: Caren Erlichman
Production Coordinator: Pamela Milcos
Compositor: David E. Seham Associates Inc.
Text Printer/Binder: R. R. Donnelley & Sons Company
Cover Printer: R. R. Donnelley & Sons Company

1   3   5   6   4   2

Library of Congress Cataloging-in-Publication Data

Preoperative cardiac assessment / edited by Dennis T. Mangano; with 8
contributors.
    p.   cm.—(A Society of Cardiovascular Anesthesiologists
monograph)
   Includes bibliographical references.
   ISBN 0-397-51089-6
   1. Heart—Surgery. 2. Preoperative care. I. Mangano, Dennis T.
II. Series.
   [DNLM: 1. Heart Diseases—complications. 2. Preoperative Care.
3. Risk Factors. WO 179 P9266]
RD598.3.P74   1990
617.4'12—dc20
DNLM/DLC
for Library of Congress   89–13948
                                                                CIP

The authors and publisher have exerted every effort to ensure that drug selection and dosage set forth in this text are in accord with current recommendations and practice at the time of publication. However, in view of ongoing research, changes in government regulations, and the constant flow of information relating to drug therapy and drug reactions, the reader is urged to check the package insert for each drug for any change in indications and dosage and for added warnings and precautions. This is particularly important when the recommended agent is a new or infrequently employed drug.

Publication Committee of the
Society of Cardiovascular Anesthesiologists

Contributors

Philip G. Boysen, MD
Professor of Medicine and
  Anesthesia
Chief, Respiratory Therapy
University of Florida College of
  Medicine
Gainesville, Florida

Paul R. Hickey, MD
Department of Anesthesia
Boston Children's Hospital
Boston, Massachusetts

John M. Jackson, MD
Assistant Professor
Department of Anesthesiology
Mayo Clinic
Minneapolis, Minnesota

Patti S. Klein, MD
Department of Anesthesia
Boston Children's Hospital
Boston, Massachusetts

Dennis T. Mangano, PhD, MD
Professor and Vice Chairman
Department of Anesthesia
University of California—San
  Francisco
San Francisco, California

Robert G. Merin, MD
Professor of Anesthesia
Department of Anesthesia
University of Texas Medical School at
  Houston
Houston, Texas

Susan Streitz, MD
Assistant in Anesthesia
Boston Children's Hospital;
Instructor in Anesthesia
Harvard Medical School
Boston, Massachusetts

Stephen J. Thomas, MD
Associate Professor
Vice Chairman and Director of
  Cardiac Thoracic Services
Department of Anesthesiology
New York Hospital—Cornell
  Medical Center
New York, New York

Contents

1

Preoperative Assessment of the Patient
with Ischemic Heart Disease
   Dennis T. Mangano

1

2

Preoperative Assessment of the Patient
with Valvular Heart Disease
   John M. Jackson
   Patti S. Klein
   Stephen J. Thomas

57

3

Preoperative Assessment of the Patient
with Congenital Heart Disease
   Paul R. Hickey
   Susan Streitz

85

4

Preoperative Assessment of the Patient
Undergoing Noncardiac Thoracic Surgery
   Philip G. Boysen

125

5 141

Preoperative Cardiovascular Medications

Robert G. Merin

Index 167

Preface

Despite major advances in diagnosis and therapeutics, cardiovascular disease remains a globally important health-care problem. One million of two million deaths annually in the United States are related to cardiovascular disease, twice the number attributable to cancer (500,000 deaths per year). Morbidity also is high, with 1.5 million myocardial infarctions, 600,000 strokes, and 400,000 cases of new congestive heart failure reported yearly. In addition, 25 million of our population is now older than 65 years, and 60 million will be over 65 in 40 years. Since the incidence of cardiovascular disease increases with age, the prevalence, intensity, mortality, and costs associated with cardiovascular disease can be expected to increase in synchrony with aging.

The impact of cardiovascular disease is substantial in patients presenting for anesthesia and surgery. Approximately 3 million of 25 million patients undergoing surgery have coronary artery disease or two or more major risk factors for coronary artery disease, and an additional 4 million are 65 years or older. Perioperative cardiac morbidity is high, and increased perioperative risk persists in those with recent myocardial infarction, congestive heart failure, symptomatic valvular disease, and several forms of congenital heart disease. Perioperative care thus remains a challenge. The cornerstone of perioperative care is the preoperative assessment of patients for anesthesia and surgery. Only by identifying at-risk patients and the severity of their diseases can we judiciously assign optimal preoperative treatment, anesthetic management techniques, and intraoperative monitoring strategies, and anticipate potential intraoperative therapeutic requirements and the need for postoperative intensive care.

Preoperative assessment of the patient with cardiovascular disease can be difficult for at least two reasons. First, the at-risk patient can be complex, presenting with a spectrum of symptoms and varying degrees of ventricular dysfunction. Second, we are in an age of cost containment, when patients present on the morning of surgery, leaving little time for evaluation. Therefore, preoperative assessment must be efficient, requiring a thorough knowledge of cardiovascular disease states, the available preoperative cardiovascular performance tests and the data they provide, and the potential perioperative risk factors.

The first 3 chapters of this monograph discuss preoperative assessment strategies for patients with ischemic heart disease, valvular heart disease, and congenital heart disease. Because of the close association between cardiovascular disease and pulmonary disease, we also present the preoperative considerations for patients with pulmonary disease in Chapter 4. Finally, in Chapter 5, we review current preoperative cardiovascular medications, highlighting newer developments and controversial regimens.

We gratefully acknowledge Winifred von Ehrenburg, Corbin Krug, and Thea Miller for their editorial assistance.

Dennis T. Mangano, PhD, MD

Preoperative Cardiac Assessment

Dennis T. Mangano

1 | Preoperative Assessment of the Patient with Ischemic Heart Disease

Between two and three million patients with coronary artery disease (CAD) or two or more major risk factors for CAD undergo anesthesia and surgery every year. Perioperative morbidity and mortality for this patient population remain high, as do costs of treating morbid complications ($12,000 per patient annually).[1] Risk factors, such as previous myocardial infarction (MI) and underlying disease requiring vascular surgery result in a 2% to 37% and 3% to 20% incidence, respectively, of current perioperative MI.[2–13] Approximately 50,000 patients per year sustain a perioperative MI, with mortality exceeding 20,000.[2–13] This problem of perioperative MI is likely to be exacerbated over the next several decades because of our aging population and the increased use of complex surgery in these higher risk patients.

The approach to perioperative morbidity has been to introduce increasingly sophisticated perioperative diagnostic and therapeutic techniques, such as preoperative exercise,[14] dipyridamole thallium-201 testing,[5] intraoperative peripheral and pulmonary artery monitoring,[7] multiple-lead electrocardiographic monitoring,[16–18] precordial and transesophageal echocardiography,[19] extended postoperative care,[7] and prophylactic therapy.[20] Although these techniques help to identify specific patient populations, they may be too costly to apply to large groups of at-risk patients. However, identification of populations at risk and preoperative assessment of their disease using routine and nonroutine tests are the cornerstones of anesthetic management.

In this chapter, we will address preoperative assessment of the cardiac patient by describing the characteristics of both preoperative routine and nonroutine cardiac tests. Anesthesiologists often discuss, interpret, or request these tests before anesthesia and should, therefore, have a knowledge of each, the specific information each provides, and the application of this information to preoperative assessment of patients with cardiac disease.

ROUTINE DIAGNOSTIC TESTS

Clinical History

Pre-existing Preoperative Syndromes

Chest pain or discomfort is a major manifestation of effort-related and at-rest angina, but is also a manifestation of such diverse clinical conditions as mitral valve prolapse, esophageal reflux, esophageal spasm, peptic ulcer disease, biliary disease, cervical disease, hyperventilation, musculoskeletal disease, and pulmonary disease. Classically, anginal pain lasts from 5 minutes to 15 minutes, with longer durations suggestive of unstable angina or MI. Briefer periods of pain—for example, transient sharp or stabbing pain—suggest other etiologies, such as musculoskeletal or gastrointestinal disorders. Anginal pain usually is related to effort, emotion, or eating, but also results from increasing myocardial oxygen consumption, such as occurs with fever, hypoglycemia, or exposure to cold. The pain associated with variant angina pectoris usually occurs at rest and is unrelated to physical exertion or emotional stress. Because the syndromes of stable, unstable, and variant angina may carry different perioperative prognoses, it is necessary to diagnose them accurately. Stable angina is a substernal discomfort precipitated by exertion and relieved by rest or nitroglycerin therapy in less than 15 minutes. Pain typically radiates to the shoulder, the jaw, or the inner aspect of the arm, but also may be isolated to these sites or to the upper abdomen. Stable angina is highly specific and sensitive for patients with coronary artery disease (CAD),[21] indicating that they may be at higher risk of developing cardiac complications (sudden death, MI) than the general population. Surprisingly, the role of stable angina in perioperative risk of complications has been denied.[22] The pattern and severity of stable angina, however, have not been isolated for study as potential risk factors.

Unstable angina is defined as: (1) new onset angina, occurring within the past 2 months; (2) progressively worsening, or at-rest, angina (occurring with increased frequency, intensity, or duration and less responsive to treatment); or (3) angina lasting longer than 30 minutes that is transiently unresponsive to standard therapeutic maneuvers (including nitroglycerin administration and rest) and is associated with transient ST- or T-wave changes, without development of Q waves or elevated enzyme levels.[23] Unstable angina may place a patient at higher risk of developing perioperative complications, but definitive information of its role in this risk is lacking.

Variant angina pectoris[24] usually occurs at rest, is unrelated to exercise or emotional stress, and is accompanied by ST-segment elevation. The perioperative risk in patients with variant angina is unknown. However, since this syndrome is associated with a greater incidence of dysrhythmias and conduction abnormalities, it is probable that patients with variant angina have a higher incidence of perioperative cardiac morbidity than those without cardiac disease.

Another syndrome devoid of clinical symptoms, silent myocardial ischemia, recently has emerged as a significant risk factor. Now recognized as a frequent and potentially serious marker of morbidity, studies of silent myocardial ischemia show that 20% to 30% of asymptomatic patients who have a myocardial infarction reveal silent ischemia on exercise stress testing postinfarction.[25] Other studies, using frequency-modulated ambulatory electrocardiographic (ECG) ST-segment monitoring, report that up to 75% of episodes of significant ST depression occur without angina and at significantly lower heart rates than symptomatic episodes.[26] In contrast, such silent ischemic episodes are rare in control groups of normal subjects.[27]

The mechanism for silent ischemia and infarction is unknown. Sensory neuropathy has been postulated, particularly in diabetics, but has not been substantiated.[28-31] Silent episodes appear to be associated with important physiologic changes. Using positron emission tomography with rubidium-82, Deanfield and colleagues found that coronary blood flow decreased significantly during episodes of asymptomatic ST depression.[32] ECG and autopsy studies show that subendocardial and transmural ischemia and MI can occur without symptoms, especially in patients with diabetes mellitus.[33-38] Although the perioperative incidence of silent ischemia is unknown, we do know that the majority of postoperative infarctions are painless.

Thus, the postoperative presence of silent myocardial ischemia may be a reliable and significant indicator of morbid outcome.

Pre-existing Medications

A history of previous and present cardiac medications and the rationales for their use should be obtained from all patients. Continuation of these medications, preoperative preparation, and intra- and postoperative anesthetic management of the patient should be based on this history of medications. The arguments for and against maintaining cardioactive medications are varied.

Assessment of Left Ventricular Function

Clinical or radiologic evidence of left ventricular (LV) failure in patients with CAD is associated with a negative prognosis[39] of increased long- and short-term morbidity and mortality. Preoperatively, an ejection fraction of less than 0.40, and dyssynergy are predictive of perioperative right and left ventricular dysfunction.[40] Thus, preoperative evidence of ventricular dysfunction increases a patient's risk of perioperative morbidity and mortality. The symptomatology can be classified using the New York Heart Association's and the Canadian Cardiovascular Society's scoring systems.[40a] Ventricular dysfunction is associated with symptoms of angina (ischemic LV paralysis). With ischemia, incomplete systolic relaxation of the myocardial fibers increases wall tension and intracardiac pressure and, therefore, pulmonary transudation pressure, which may result in transient symptoms of congestive heart failure. Though transient, the latter symptoms are a significant finding, because they may substantially increase the patient's perioperative risk and thus warrant more invasive monitoring of intracardiac pressures.

The Physical Examination

In addition to manifest signs of left or right ventricular failure, there are other important preoperative signs of perioperative risk. In patients with CAD, a displaced point of maximal impulse caused, for example, by cardiomegaly, usually indicates that the ejection fraction is less than 50%, which places the patient at increased risk.[39,40] With prior MI, an abnormal precordial systolic bulge may occur, indicating an LV wall-motion abnormality, which is also predictive of perioperative ventricular dysfunction.[41] Altered ventricular compliance can be associated with a fourth heart sound, common in patients with CAD, especially in the presence of a prior MI or acute angina. Third heart sounds are associated with elevation of the LV end-diastolic pressure, usually with a prior extensive MI. Both third and fourth heart sounds appear to be related to hemodynamic and ventriculographic findings in patients with CAD. For example, Cohn and coworkers[42] found, by using phonocardiogram, that 42 of 93 patients with CAD had third or fourth heart sounds. The incidence of these heart sounds appears to increase with stress (hand-grip exercise),[43] unstable angina,[44] and exercise.[45] They have important diagnostic value, but the specific interpretation of these heart sounds can be difficult,[46] particularly in elderly patients. For example, the finding of an apical systolic murmur, without other signs of valvular heart disease, may indicate papillary muscle dysfunction associated with prior MI or acute angina pectoris. Finally, the presence of conditions such as rales, cardiomegaly, jugular venous distension, and pulmonary edema also increase the patient's risk of morbid perioperative outcome.[47]

Laboratory Tests

Most preoperative laboratory test data are normal in patients with CAD. Hyperlipidemia or carbohydrate intolerance, however, are predictive of CAD and are related to coronary angiographic findings.[48] They are therefore useful in identifying patients who may be at risk of morbid cardiac outcome. An increase in low-density lipoproteins (types 2 or 4) appears to be a strong predictor of CAD, whereas a high-density lipoprotein:cholesterol ratio appears to correlate with protection from CAD. Triglyceride levels appear to be relatively unimportant predictors of CAD.[49] Increased platelet aggregation during exercise-induced myocardial ischemia, however, also may identify patients with CAD.[50]

The biochemical change most often associated with myocardial ischemia and infarction is an increase in the level of cardiac enzymes. Irreversible myocardial cell damage results in elevated levels of creatine kinase (CK), glutamic oxaloacetic transferase (GOT), and lactate dehydrogenase (LD). GOT levels usually increase above the normal range within 8 to 12 hours after the onset of chest pain, with peak levels occurring 18 to 36 hours after infarction, and return to normal within 3 to 4 days (Fig. 1-1). CK levels rise above normal approximately 6 to 8 hours after infarction, peak at 24 hours, and return to

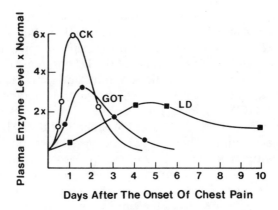

FIGURE 1-1. Typical plasma concentrations of cardiac enzymes following the onset of chest pain associated with acute myocardial infarction. *CK* = creatine kinase, *GOT* = glutamic oxaloacetic transferase, and *LD* = lactic dehydrogenase.
(Hearse DJ: Myocardial enzyme leakage. J Mol Med 2:185, 1977)

normal within 3 to 4 days. The isoenzymes of CK (MM, BB, and MB), identified by electrophoresis, differentiate tissue extraction from brain and kidney (BB), skeletal muscle (MM), and cardiac muscle (MB). CK–MB levels are a highly specific (greater than 90%) and reasonably sensitive indicator (greater than 65%) of acute MI. Prediction of infarct size from serial measurements of CK–MB also appears to be reasonably accurate.[51–53] LD increases above the normal range between 24 and 48 hours after acute MI, peaks between 3 and 6 days, and returns to normal after 8 to 14 days. GOT and LD are sensitive, but not specific, enzymes, resulting in false positive readings in patients with noncardiac diseases. However, the first isoenzyme of LD, LD_1, occurs principally in the heart and rises above normal 8 to 24 hours after infarction. The ratio of LD_1 to LD is abnormal in 95% of patients with acute MI.[52,54]

Electrocardiography

The resting electrocardiogram (ECG) is normal in 25% to 50% of patients with CAD[55] and is probably nondiagnostic in an additional 25% because of conditions such as left bundle branch block or Wolff–Parkinson–White syndrome. Despite this, the ECG is one of the most important preoperative tests for patients with CAD. Patterns of ischemia, injury and infarction, conduction changes, and dysrhythmias may have important prognostic significance.

Characteristic patterns describing ischemia, injury, and infarction in animals with acute coronary ligation, show a T wave that peaks, followed by ST elevation. The polarity of the T wave remains upright in humans with subendocardial ischemia because the direction of repolarization is undisturbed, proceeding from epicardium to endocardium. In contrast, the T wave is inverted during subepicardial ischemia, because the direction of repolarization is reversed from endocardium to epicardium. Recovery may be prolonged in such cases, resulting in larger, elongated T waves. With myocardial injury, either diastolic or systolic currents of injury may occur. With diastolic currents of injury, the PQ segment is deflected downward and, despite its isoelectricity, the ST segment is elevated relative to the depressed baseline. With systolic currents of injury, no baseline (PQ) abnormality occurs, but the injured area repolarizes more rapidly, resulting in ST elevation. Subendocardial injury is detected as ST-segment elevation if the sensing electrode faces the endocardium, or as ST-segment depression if the sensing electrode faces the normal epicardium. With subepicardial injury, the opposite occurs.

MI is classically detected by the presence of a Q wave if the infarction is transmural, or persistent ST elevation for several days if the infarction is subendocardial. The sequence of ECG changes with MI appears to be similar in both human and animal models. The earliest change is a T-wave abnormality, with the T wave either prolonged or magnified, and either upright or inverted.[56,57] ST-segment elevation occurs in the leads facing the injured area, and reciprocal ST-segment depression occurs in those facing away from the injured area. Significant Q waves (greater than 0.04 seconds and ⅓ of the height of the R wave) may develop soon thereafter, after a period of days, or never. R-wave amplitude may decrease during infarction. Finally, the ST segment becomes isoelectric and the T wave becomes symmetrically inverted.[58]

This classic sequence occurs in approximately 50% to 70% of patients sustaining an MI[59,60] and is highly specific for the diagnosis of an acute MI. In the remainder of patients, ST- and T-wave changes may be the only manifestation. The more difficult clinical questions occur when nonspecific ST-segment and T-wave changes appear on the ECG. Early, marked ST-segment changes (greater than 2 mm) are highly specific for myocardial injury. However, these changes must persist for a period of days for a diagnosis of infarction. Other conditions are associated with transient, marked ST elevation or depression, such as Prinzmetal's angina, pericarditis, ventricular aneurysm, and subendocardial injury. Pseudonormalization of T waves and even ST segments may occur during a true infarction process, confounding the diagnosis.

Chest Radiography

In patients with CAD, the chest radiograph can provide useful information about ventricular function. Four radiographic indices are specific indicators of abnormal ventricular function.[22] The cardiothoracic ratio, total heart volume, LV volume, and signs of congestive heart failure are specific indicators of abnormal ejection fraction, end-systolic volume, cardiac index, stroke work index, end-diastolic volume and end-diastolic pressure. The relatively high specificities (68%–72%) of the radiographic indices indicate that abnormal results in a patient with CAD identify abnormal ventricular function. For example, cardiomegaly predicts a low ejection fraction. Normal radiographic results, however, do not preclude ventricular dysfunction. A normal heart size may be associated with normal or abnormal function. The routine preoperative chest radiograph thus provides significant information only when function is abnormal. MI cannot be detected using the chest radiograph unless it is associated with a large aneurysm or significant calcification.[61,62] Finally, visualization of calcium deposits within the coronary arteries, although useful, is difficult using chest radiography.

NONROUTINE DIAGNOSTIC TESTS

Exercise Stress Testing

Exercise-induced changes in cardiac performance were first detected on the ECG by Einthoven in 1908.[63] Both P wave and T wave amplitude and heart rate increased with stair climbing. A relationship between angina pectoris and the ECG was established[64] when ST-T abnormalities were found to be associated with at-rest angina, as well as exercise-induced angina. A two-step exercise technique was developed[65] and tested in patients with angina pectoris,[66] resulting in standardization of exercise stress testing for this patient population. Relatively recent protocols include the bicycle ergometer and the treadmill. The major differences between exercise stress-testing protocols are the grade, speed, and duration of each stage of the test. The predictive value of this testing technique for CAD is controversial. In this section, we will discuss the physiology, types of exercise tests, the ST-segment response, other outcomes, and indications and conclusions.

Exercise stress testing appears to be relatively safe. Rochmis and Blackburn[67] surveyed 73 exercise stress-testing laboratories and found 16 deaths in 170,000 tests. Forty additional patients had nonfatal complications requiring hospitalization. The mortality appears to be approximately 1 in 10,000, and morbidity is approximately 4 in 10,000.

All exercise stress test protocols progressively increase myocardial work while measuring the signs and symptoms of ischemia, dysrhythmia, and ventricular dysfunction. Exercise generally is induced using treadmills, bicycles, or isometric techniques in noninvasive cardiac catheterization or radionuclear laboratories. Outcomes usually are assessed clinically and electrocardiographically. In select circumstances, ventricular function data are obtained using ventriculography or radionuclear imaging. Familiar treadmill protocols are those introduced by Bruce,[68] Ellestad,[69] Astrand,[70] and Sheffield,[71] some of which are shown in Figure 1-2. In each of these protocols, exercise is performed in stages defined by treadmill speed and grade and lasts from 1 minute to 10 or more minutes. The most familiar of these, the Bruce protocol,[68] consists of 3-minute stages that differ in both grade and speed. Stage 1 has a speed of 1.7 mph with a 10% grade, and stage 5 (12 to 15 minutes) has a speed of 5 mph with an 18% grade. Patients with moderate coronary disease typically exercise to stages 3 and 4 before termination of the test because of symptoms or heart-rate limitations. Well-trained athletes (marathon athletes) are able to exercise to stages 7 or 8 before exhaustion occurs. Studies comparing blood pressure, heart rate, and oxygen uptake results for these tests have found no significant differences; however, difficulties in the performances of these tests exist for patients with impaired cardiac function.

The ST-Segment Response

During exercise and the immediate recovery period, the principal indicator of myocardial ischemia is ECG ST-segment deviation. During early-stage exercise, heart rate increases and the J point of the ST

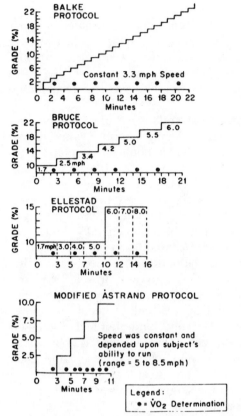

FIGURE 1-2. Four exercise stress test protocols demonstrating differences in grade, speed, stage duration, and oxygen consumption determinations. *(Pollock ML et al: A comparative analysis of four protocols for maximal treadmill stress testing. Am Heart J 92:39, 1976)*

segment becomes depressed. However, the slope of the ST segment rises and merges with the T wave. This response occurs in normal individuals and in patients with CAD. With endocardial ischemia, the diastolic injury potential vector opposes that of the QRS complex, and ST-segment depression deflects downward, with a slope equal to or less than 0 (flat or downsloping). Downward ST-segment deflection having this slope is considered consistent with ischemia. The magnitude of the ST depression also is important. Although depressions of 1 mm (0.1 millivolts) are the accepted threshold for diagnosis of ischemia, the criteria for interpreting the magnitude of ST depression differ by the lead system used, and the desired degree of sensitivity and specificity. For example, choosing 0.5 mm as the criterion minimizes false negatives (high sensitivity), but produces many false positives (low specificity); in contrast, 2 mm is a highly specific index having low sensitivity. Bipolar lead systems, for example, are more sensitive than unipolar systems, and some use a 2 mm deflection criterion. Thus, reported criteria vary and must be interpreted carefully.

Three types of ST-segment exercise and postexercise responses have been described.[71] The first type is characterized by an ST depression with a flat or downsloping segment during the exercise period, which reverts to normal soon after exercise. This response is considered severe when: the magnitude of the depression is greater than 2 mm; depression occurs during the early stages (1–3) of the test; or, hypotension occurs during the exercise period. During the second type, the ST depression worsens during the recovery period and is associated with a poor prognosis. The third type of ST response is ST-segment elevation, reportedly occurring in approximately 5% of patients undergoing stress testing. The conventionally accepted criterion is a threshold of elevation of 1.5 mm or more, regardless of slope. This type of response can be associated with fixed coronary lesions, with scarring or dyskinesia due to previous infarction, or with coronary spasm (Prinzmetal's variant angina). Although variant angina usually occurs at rest, exercise stress testing may precipitate this response.

Prognostically, it appears that the ST-segment response is most predictive in at-risk populations who demonstrate significant and early changes during stress testing. In patients with coronary risk factors, the sensitivity of exercise stress testing is approximately 70% and the specificity is about 90%. With significant exercise or postexercise ST depression, the incidence of coronary events increases threefold to sevenfold within 1 to 5 years after the test.[68,72,73] In asymptomatic patients, exercise stress testing is less useful. In one study,[73] 75 of 2,014 healthy men had ST depression of at least 1.5 mm; of these 75, 48 had anatomic CAD evidenced by arteriography. Although this represents a predictive value of 64% and identifies a patient population at risk, the Seattle Heart Watch Group found that exercise stress testing offered no prognostic advantage in asymptomatic individuals without coronary risk factors.[68]

The severity and onset of ST depression appear to correlate with anatomic disease. ST depression of 1 mm to 3 mm or more occurring during stages 2 or 3 of a Bruce protocol is associated with a 67% probability of 1- to 3-vessel disease. Changes of 2 mm or more occurring during stages 1 or 2 are associated with a 90% probability of 1- to 3-vessel disease. Among patients with ST depression of 3 mm or more, Goldman and colleagues[74] found that 69% had 3-vessel disease and 92% had left anterior descending disease.

The early occurrence of ST changes (stage 1 or stage 2) is associated with a poor prognosis. Among patients who developed significant (2 mm or more) ST depression during stage 1 of the Bruce protocol, 40% had cardiac events during the first year following exercise stress testing.[75-77] The test has limitations, however. Assessing the location of anatomic lesions from exercise stress test lead information is difficult. More importantly, negative test results do not exclude the presence of disease. Approximately one third of the patients undergoing coronary artery bypass graft surgery with demonstrable anatomic lesions have negative exercise stress-testing results.

Additional Responses

Changes in the T wave or R wave, the occurrence of chest pain, altered heart rate, hypotension, or dysrhythmias also indicate patients at risk of perioperative morbidity. Symmetrical T-wave inversion usually is associated with CAD, but is generally considered a nonspecific sign during exercise stress testing because of its association with hypertension, electrolyte disturbances, and cardiomyopathy. The QRS magnitude may be a function of the intracavity LV volume (the Brody effect).[78] R-wave amplitude increases with increasing intraventricular volume. In patients with CAD and incomplete systolic emptying (increased end-systolic volume), there is often increased R-wave amplitude, which may be associated with myocardial ischemia. Using a bipolar lead system, Bonoris and colleagues[79,80] found that R-wave amplitude remained the same or increased in patients with CAD, but decreased in normal patients. Both the specificity and sensitivity of the bipolar system increased when R-wave amplitude, rather than ST-segment deflection, was used as a measure of myocardial ischemia. Hollenberg and coworkers[81] found that the prognostic value of the ST segment can be increased by incorporating R wave amplitude into the normalization of the ST segment response.

The occurrence of angina during exercise stress testing increases the prognostic value of the ST response. Ellestad[69] found that when the ST response was associated with angina, negative outcome events increased twofold over the four-year period following the study. The early occurrence of angina also has prognostic significance. Patients with angina occurring early at four METS had twice the rate of events as patients expending twice this energy later in the test.* Hemody-

---

*1 MET = 3.5 ml of oxygen consumed per kilogram of body weight per minute.

namic changes in heart rate and blood pressure offer additional prognostic value. Even without an ST-segment response, a subnormal heart rate response may be as predictive as the ST response itself.[69] A subnormal blood pressure response (less than 30 mm Hg during stages 2 or 3) markedly enhances the prognostic value of the ST response. For example, 77% of patients with exertional hypotension had significant left main or left main equivalent disease.[82]

For the detection of dysrhythmias, exercise stress testing increases the yield of premature ventricular contractions threefold over the resting ECG and eightfold for repetitive forms of ventricular dysrhythmias. Approximately 52% of patients with CAD exhibit premature ventricular contractions during exercise stress testing. The contractions usually occur, not only at peak exercise, but also during the initial 3 minutes of recovery; in fact, ventricular fibrillation most commonly occurs during the recovery period.

Indications and Conclusions. Exercise stress testing is a relatively inexpensive, noninvasive test useful in diagnosing patients with chest pain of unknown etiology and in quantifying CAD and determining prognosis in patients with CAD. Exercise stress testing has significant prognostic value when the characteristic ST changes have significant magnitude (greater than 1.5 mm), occur during early stages of the test (stages 1–3), are sustained into the recovery period, are associated with subnormal increases in heart rate or blood pressure, and are accompanied by angina or dysrhythmias. It appears to have limited value, however, as a generalized screening procedure in healthy, asymptomatic patients.

As a preoperative screening test, exercise stress testing is useful for defining new-onset, atypical chest pain. If this unstable angina is indicative of ischemia, perioperative morbidity and mortality may be markedly increased. The angina may develop a crescendo characteristic or may reflect the early stage of infarction. The chest pain pattern must be defined, and appropriate medical therapy must begin prior to anesthesia and surgery.

Several exercise stress test results are especially important to the anesthesiologist, the first being the diagnosis of CAD. It is useful to know the magnitude of the ST-response changes, the onset and duration of these changes, and the associated hemodynamic effects. The therapies used during exercise stress testing to reverse ischemia also may be useful for intraoperative treatment of ischemic changes. Dysrhythmias occurring during exercise or the recovery period indicate and suggest treatment for perioperative dysrhythmias. The heart rate and blood pressure at which ischemic events occur may serve as guidelines for perioperative control of these variables.

Echocardiography

Echocardiography has become an important noninvasive method of assessing regional wall motion and wall thickening, global ventricular function, valvular function, and coronary anatomy. The principle of echocardiography is based on the detection of sound waves reflected from the surfaces of internal organs. In comparison with the audible sound range (20 to 20,000 Hz), frequencies used in echocardiography range from 1 to 7 MHz. At the higher frequencies (5–7 MHz), resolutions of 1 mm are possible, but penetration of surface structures decreases with increasing frequency. The lower frequencies (1–3 MHz) produce lower resolution (2–3 mm), but better penetration. For precordial echocardiography, frequencies of 2 to 3 MHz are used, which allow 2 mm resolution and penetration of the chest wall. With transesophageal echocardiography, penetration is not difficult, permitting the use of higher frequencies (3.5–5 MHz) that achieve excellent resolutions. Significant advances of the last decade include the refinement of M-mode echocardiography and the introduction of two-dimensional, Doppler color-flow and, most recently, contrast echocardiography. In this section, we review these advances and discuss the uses of echocardiography for detection of wall-motion and wall-thickening abnormalities and for determination of global ventricular function.

M-Mode Echocardiography

A typical M-mode echocardiogram is shown in Figure 1-3. With the transducer placed on the chest wall, the M-mode (one-dimensional mode) represents an "ice-pick" view of the heart. The tracing represents this one-dimensional view plotted against time. Systolic and diastolic events can be visualized in a single dimension or in multiple dimensions by redirecting the transducer along several lines through the heart. With the patient in the left lateral decubitus position, the transducer is swept along the left parasternal border from the level of the aortic valve to the LV cavity. The motion of valves and walls and the linear dimensions of intracardiac and pericardiac structures can be visualized. These views permit linear estimates of end-diastolic and end-systolic LV dimensions and calculations of ejection

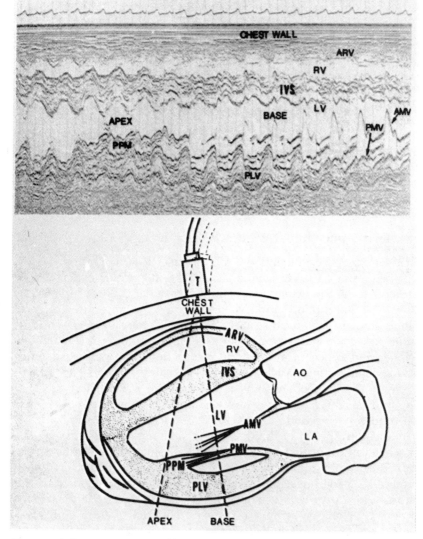

FIGURE 1-3. Typical M-mode echocardiogram of the left ventricle with a pictorial display. The transducer is swept from base to apex at the level of the posterior papillary muscle. With systolic contraction the posterior papillary muscle and posterior left ventricular wall move toward the interventricular septum. *AMV* = anterior mitral valve leaflet; *AO* = aorta; *ARV* = anterior right ventricular wall; *IVS* = interventricular septum; *LA* = left atrium; *LV* = left ventricle; *PLV* = posterior left ventricular wall; *PMV* = posterior mitral valve leaflet; *RV* = right ventricle; *PPM* = posterior papillary muscle; *T* = transducer. *(Corya BC: Applications of echocardiography in acute myocardial infarction. Cardiovasc Clin 2:113, 1975)*

fraction and fiber shortening. Wall-motion and wall-thickening abnormalities can be estimated as well.

M-mode echocardiography has limited value in patients with CAD who have segmental wall-motion abnormalities (dyssynergy). Although estimates for a given segment will accurately reflect localized changes, they cannot be used to estimate global function because other normal contracting and hypercontracting segments will exist and be undetected. Thus, M-mode linear dimension estimates of intracardiac volumes and ejection fractions are unreliable in this patient population. Despite these limitations, M-mode echocardiography is valuable for diagnosis of a number of other disease states.

Two-Dimensional Echocardiography

Real time cross-sectional, two-dimensional echocardiography was developed from M-mode echocardiography. It enables evaluation of structures perpendicular to the unidimensional beam, characterization of lateral motion, and visual integration of an entire sector of single-dimensional beams. A typical two-dimensional echocardiogram using the parasternal long-axis view is shown in Figure 1-4. While M-mode echocardiography records temporal perturbations of any structure lying parallel to its beam, two-dimensional echocardiography simultaneously scans an entire sector of the field by recording individual b-mode lines on videotape at a sampling rate of 30 to 60 frames per second (versus 1,000 impulses per second with M-mode). With the tip of the transducer stationary, the beam is either mechanically moved through an arc by using an oscillating single transducer or by rotating a series of transducers, or it is steered electronically, using phased-array ultrasonic elements that constitute the beam. These scanners usually are referred to as mechanical sector scanners or phased-array scanners.[83,84] The images from both scanners are similar, and both techniques are undergoing rather rapid technological changes.

Two-dimensional echocardiography enables the recording of lateral wall motion, axial motion, and multiple planes. The most common planes visualized are the parasternal long-axis view, the short-axis view at the level of the mitral valve and the papillary muscle, and the apical and four-chamber views. In any of these views, wall motion and wall thickening during systole and diastole can be quantified, and end-diastolic and end-systolic areas can be estimated. Echocardiographic measures of global ventricular function correlate well

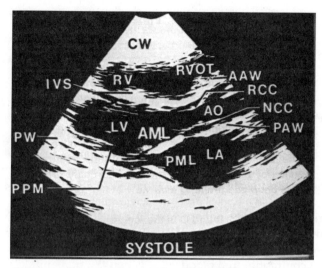

FIGURE 1-4.   Typical two-dimensional echocardiogram illustration demonstrating the parasternal long-axis view of the heart in systole. *AAW* = anterior aortic wall; *AML* = anterior mitral leaflet; *AO* = aorta; *CW* = chest wall; *IVS* = interventricular septum; *LA* = left atrium; *LV* = left ventricle; *NCC* = noncoronary cusp; *PAW* = posterior aortic wall; *PML* = posterior mitral leaflet; *PPM* = posteromedial papillary muscle; *PW* = posterior wall (left ventricle); *RCC* = right coronary cusp; *RV* = right ventricle; *RVOT* = right ventricular outflow tract. *(Talano JV: Cardiac Ultrasound Workbook. New York, Grune & Stratton, 1982)*

(r = 0.75 or greater) with radiographic and angiographic data. Multiple plane views are necessary, however, for accurate estimates of these measurements.[85,86]

Transesophageal Two-Dimensional Echocardiography

Transesophageal echocardiography is a technique developed in Europe during the last decade that is used in both anesthetized and awake (lightly sedated) patients. A 9-mm gastroscope with a transducer placed at its distal end is passed into the esophagus and advanced to obtain aortic valve, four-chamber, mitral valve (papillary muscle), and apical views of the heart. Because the transducer is nearly in direct contact with the heart and sound waves do not have to penetrate the chest wall or lung structures, higher frequency transducers (3.5–5 MHz) enable 1-mm resolution and very high-quality images.

Doppler Echocardiography

Doppler echocardiography is based on the physical characteristics of sound waves: When a sound wave of a particular frequency is transmitted and reflected off a moving object, the frequency difference between the transmitted and reflected waves is proportional to the velocity of the moving object and the angle at which the transmitted wave strikes the object. Given this angle and the Doppler shift frequency difference, the velocity of the moving object can be calculated. It is possible to calculate velocities of cardiac valves, ventricular walls and, most commonly, red blood cells. When the transmitted signal is a continuous wave, the technique is referred to as "continuous-wave" Doppler. Using continuous-wave Doppler, blood flow can be quantified accurately in superficial arteries and veins[87–90] and can be estimated in central arteries like the aorta or common carotid artery. Absolute values for central blood flow are more difficult to obtain, although accuracy appears to be improving with newer techniques.

The most recent advances in Doppler technology incorporate continuous-wave Doppler with the pulsed ultrasound technique used for cardiac imaging. Using this combination, cardiac structures can be imaged, flows across these structures can be quantified, and valve orifice size can be estimated. Because the Doppler shift is in the audible range, Doppler echocardiography can enhance clinical diagnosis. In addition, from time-interval histogram displays, laminar flow can be distinguished from turbulent flow through or across intracardiac structures, such as valves. With laminar flow, the detected velocities are approximately equal; with turbulent flow, however, Doppler signals are scattered and represent a combination of multiple velocities and directions of flow.

Doppler technology is improving rapidly. A number of technical problems exist, such as aliasing with pulsed Doppler, spatial localization with continuous-wave Doppler, and quantifying velocities with both techniques. Intraoperative Doppler echocardiography, using a precordial or transesophageal approach, offers significant potential for characterizing the dynamic state of the circulation.

Contrast Echocardiography

Injection of a liquid into the circulation creates microbubbles that can be visualized using echocardiography. Intra-atrial and ventricular septal defects producing right-to-left shunts have been diagnosed using this form of contrast echocardiography. Various contrast agents have been used, including saline, dye, carbon dioxide, and hydrogen peroxide. This technique is gaining in popularity and may offer significant potential for visualizing intracardiac and, possibly, coronary artery structures. Significant advances should be made over the next 5 years.

Intraoperatively, this technique has been used to identify patients with right-to-left shunts, which is especially useful during sitting craniotomies. Several preliminary reports have demonstrated that contrast echocardiography enables visualization of septal defects using the transesophageal approach, making it potentially useful as a monitor in such situations.

Visualization of Coronary Arteries. During the past decade, a group of investigators has used echocardiography to identify coronary arteries. Block and Popp[91] adequately visualized the coronary arteries in 37 of 50 patients, and correctly identified left main CAD in 4 of 5 patients. Future refinements, such as strobe freeze-frame analysis, digital gray-scale analysis, and advanced signal processing,[91-93] will extend the use of this technique even more.

Evaluation of Wall Motion and Wall Thickening. Studies in animals have demonstrated that, soon after coronary occlusion, the ischemic myocardium develops wall-motion and wall-thickening abnormalities. Two-dimensional echocardiography appears to have a significant advantage over M-mode echocardiography for detection of these abnormalities. With M-mode, only an "ice-pick" view of the ventricle is provided, and regions of segmental wall-motion abnormality may be missed. Two-dimensional echocardiography, however, permits qualitative and quantitative assessment of segmental wall-motion abnormalities. Qualitatively, wall motion is classified as hyperkinetic (greater than normal), normal, hypokinetic (normal direction, but reduced motion), akinetic (absent motion), or dyskinetic (paradoxic motion). Wall-motion abnormalities may be quantitated using several methods, one of which, adapted from Heger and colleagues,[94] is shown in Figure 1-5.

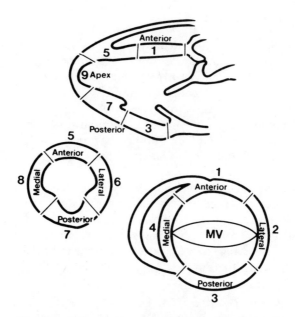

FIGURE 1-5. A typical method for defining specific left ventricular segments for wall-motion analysis. *(Heger J et al.: Cross-sectional echocardiography in acute myocardial infarction: Detection and localization of regional left ventricular asynergy. Circulation 60:531, 1979)*

In this commonly used method, the ventricle is divided into nine segments of approximately equal size, and the segments are defined according to fixed anatomic landmarks. For each segment, wall motion can be quantified by measuring the degree of radial shortening and the amount of wall thinning occurring during systole. This system classifies a segment as normal if the radius shortens by more than 30%, and wall thickening occurs with systole. Hypokinesis is radial shortening of less than 30%, also with wall thickening, whereas akinesis is radial shortening of less than 10%, without wall thickening during systole. Dyskinesis is defined by radial lengthening and wall thinning.

Segmental wall-motion abnormalities have become the standard for definition of myocardial ischemia; other factors can affect wall motion and endocardial excursion, however, and potentially confound interpretation. For example, a normal variation in the degree of endocardial excursion with systole makes absolute quantification difficult. Temperature, intracardiac volume, ventricular interference, and abnormalities of electrical conduction also may affect wall motion. Consequently, wall thickening may be a better indicator of myocardial ischemia, because it is less affected by spatial motion of the ventricle or alterations in ventricular shape. The ventricular wall thickens during systole by approximately 14% to 57% (an average of 36%).[95] Decreases in wall thickening occur with acute ischemia if there is a scar from a previous MI. Wall thinning with systole appears to occur only with acute myocardial ischemia and infarction.[96–98] Mean wall thickening decreases by approximately 50% with MI when 20% of the myocardium is infarcted, and infarctions of greater than 20% are associated with wall thinning.[99] Two-dimensional echocardiography appears to be particularly useful in detecting wall-thickening changes. In the future, improved methods of endocardial mapping using advanced data processing techniques will be used to characterize wall-thickening changes, permitting quantitative assessment of acute ischemic and infarction changes.

Global Ventricular Function. Although LV function in normal ventricles can be quantified using both M-mode and two-dimensional echocardiography, M-mode echocardiography is inaccurate in patients having ventricular dysfunction with wall-motion abnormalities. Two-dimensional echocardiography, however, can provide estimates of ejection fraction, velocity of circumferential fiber shortening, and ventricular volumes. Prerequisite are the adequate visualization of the endocardial surface, reproducible transducer positioning, and imaging of the maximum cavity size from each selected position. Within these constraints, ejection fractions and ventricular volumes can be calculated, and the values can correlate well with those derived from ventriculography or radionuclear techniques, although precise estimates are difficult to obtain from the single-plane, two-dimensional echocardiogram. Multiple planes (3–4) are necessary for relative precision.[100–102]

Echocardiographic volumes consistently underestimate true ventricular cavity volume because of endocardial interference (which broadens the echoes), failure to include the cavity volume contained within the trabeculae, artifactual diastolic or systolic reduction of wall motion through the scan plane, and other technical limitations.[103–106] In contrast, angiographically obtained volumes consistently overestimate true volume because of inclusion of papillary muscle and mitral valve apparatus in the calculations, silhouette formatting (which maximizes the projected area), and inclusion of the trabeculae. Compared with the angiographic technique, end-systolic volumes determined echocardiographically are more accurate than end-diastolic volumes because of the improved definition of the endocardial surface at end-systole. The accuracy of any quantitative ventricular function technique depends on the applied formulae, the frequency of sampling, and the configuration of the ventricle. The most accurate technique appears to follow Simpson's rule, using sections spaced 3 mm apart.

Conclusions. As a preoperative test, precordial echocardiography is a noninvasive, relatively inexpensive test that has specific advantages in several clinical situations. First, it is useful for the diagnosis of an acute MI when other techniques, such as ECG, are uninterpretable (because of left bundle branch block, Wolff–Parkinson–White syndrome). Second, for assessment of global ventricular function, two-dimensional echocardiography provides useful information on ejection fraction (correlation of 0.78 to 0.94), end-systolic and end-diastolic volumes, and circumferential wall motion and ventricular mass. This may be particularly useful in patients undergoing major third-space surgery or surgery involving aortic cross-clamping in whom the degree of ventricular dysfunction is not apparent from routine clinical test. Also, in patients with a questionable anginal pattern, wall-motion and wall-thickening changes assessed echocardiographically at rest or during exercise can provide both qualitative and quantitative information. In patients undergoing extensive surgery, this technique may be useful for deciding optimal preoperative management and perioperative monitoring and care. Finally, echocardiography is useful for definition of LV aneurysm, septal rupture, papillary muscle abnormalities, and mural thrombus formation.

Nuclear Imaging

Nuclear imaging of the cardiovascular system has advanced significantly and is now a safe and accurate method for assessing myocardial perfusion and infarction and ventricular function. One of the earliest descriptions of the use of nuclear imaging was in 1927 when radioactive radon was injected intravenously, and circulation time was measured using a modified Wilson cloud chamber.[107] Imaging of the heart using radiocardiograms was first described by Prinzmetal and coworkers.[108] Significant advances in cardiac perfusion and function measurements have been made in the last 20 years, including instrumentation, radiopharmaceuticals, and techniques for MI and perfusion imaging in the evaluation of cardiac performance.

Instrumentation

The scintillation camera, also known as the Anger or gamma camera, detects gamma rays from an injected radiopharmaceutical, converts the energy to electrical energy, and displays this representation of radioactivity. The scintillation camera consists of a collimator that absorbs gamma rays and passes them through multiple channels, or holes. The gamma rays are, in effect, focused by the collimator to a receiving crystal that converts the gamma ray energy to light. The crystal is a positron-sensitive detector made of sodium iodide. The light energy is enhanced and converted into electrical energy by photomultiplier tubes packed tightly against the crystal. The electrical signals are then electronically processed by the detector, and the energy from the original gamma rays is calculated and spatially described.

A second type of camera, the multicrystal scintillation camera, has 294 sodium iodide crystals and 35 photomultiplier tubes associated with the crystal array. Signal processing of photomultiplier row and column tubes allows spatial identification of scintillation events. Because of its design, count rates of 500,000 events per second can be recorded, so that the multicrystal camera can be used for dynamic studies, such as first-pass radionuclide angiography.

Another detector, the single-probe scintillation detector, allows measurement of ejection fraction, cardiac output, pulmonary transit time, and other measures of global LV function. Its significant advantages are that it is small and portable and can be used in a large number of environments. The actual probe is approximately 3 inches in diameter by 2 inches in depth and uses a variety of collimators. Following injection of the radiopharmaceutical, such as technetium 99m, passage through the right heart pulmonary circulation and the left heart can be recorded by measuring count rates during the systolic and diastolic cycles (first-pass angiography). The radiopharmaceuticals also may be used to label albumin or red blood cells, and the study may be gated to the ECG following equilibration (equilibration radionuclide angiography). End-systolic and end-diastolic counts, ejection fraction, cardiac output, and pulmonary transit time may be measured from the time activity curves.

Single-photon, or positron-emission, tomography—another detector—allows differentiation of myocardial regions, resolution of adjacent structures, and isolation of background noise. Both limited-angle and transaxial tomography are used, but only transaxial tomography appears to provide the required depth resolution. Positron-transaxial tomography is currently being used in studies of regional myocardial metabolism and perfusion.

Myocardial Infarction Imaging

Diagnosis of an acute MI using history and electrocardiographic and enzymatic data is not always possible, because the MI may be asymptomatic, the ECG may be uninterpretable, or cardiac enzymatic changes may be masked by other tissue effects, such as skeletal muscle destruction during surgery. Nuclear imaging techniques can help significantly to determine the presence and extent of MI.

Hot-Spot Imaging.   Two types of imaging exist for diagnosis of MI. The principal method, infarct-avid myocardial scintigraphy (hot-spot imaging), uses technetium-99m pyrophosphate as the radionuclide (technetium-pyrophosphate imaging), as the infarcted segment of the myocardium has a selective affinity for technetium. Once technetium is taken up, the increased activity of the area, referred to as a hot spot, can be detected using a gamma camera. Because normal tissue or areas of old scarring and infarction have no affinity for technetium, these areas are not visualized. The uptake in acute MI depends on the regional blood flow, the concentration of calcium in the myocardium, the reversibility of the myocardial injury, and the time of infarction. The earliest detectable images are seen from 12 to 16 hours following infarct, but maximum abnormality occurs from 48 to 72 hours afterwards. After 5 to 7 days, the intensity of the image approaches normal (Fig. 1-6).

Technetium-99m pyrophosphate is a readily available radionuclide with favorable photon energies (140 KeV) and a short halflife (6 hours). Following injection into a peripheral vein, 50% of the dose is extracted by bone and the remainder is rapidly excreted through the kidneys, with 5% of the injected dose remaining in the blood 90 minutes after injection. With acute coronary occlusion in animals, the infarcted area concentration is approximately 20 times that of normal tissue. Because a minimal coronary blood flow of 20% to 40% to the infarcted area is necessary for adequate radionuclide uptake, false negatives may occur. Additionally, endocardial concentrations appear to be significantly less than epicardial concentrations, and sub-endocardial MIs may escape detection. At least 5 grams of infarcted tissue are estimated to be necessary for adequate detection. Once the

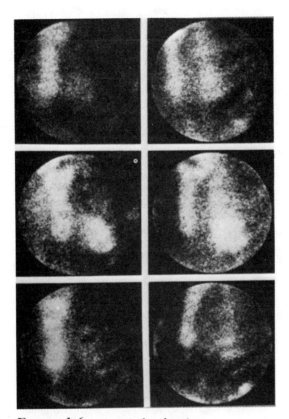

FIGURE 1-6.   A typical technetium
pyrophosphate image in a patient with an acute
transmural myocardial infarction. *(Top)* A faintly
positive image is seen lateral to the sternum over the
left ventricle, approximately 10 hours after
myocardial infarction. *(Middle)* A more intense
image, 3 days following infarction. *(Bottom)* Marked
reduction of the myocardial uptake of technetium, 7
days following infarction. *(Willerson JT, Parkey RW,
Bonte FJ et al.: Technetium stannous pyrophosphate
myocardial scintigrams in patients with chest pain of
varying etiology. Circulation 51:1046, 1975)*

isotope binds to the infarcted tissue, the radionuclide emits photons that allow detection and localization of the MI by the gamma camera. The mechanism by which the infarcted tissue binds this radioisotope is unknown, but it appears to involve myocardial calcium. Intracellular calcium deposition occurs during myocardial necrosis and may complex with the radionuclide.[109]

Technetium-pyrophosphate imaging has a greater than 90% sensitivity in the detection of acute MI.[110] Infarcts can be detected in dogs when as little as 2% of the ventricular mass is affected. There is a strong correlation between uptake technetium, infarcted areas, ECG Q waves, and myocardial perfusion defects detected scintigraphically. The determination of infarct size using this technique is under study.

Cold-Spot Imaging. A second nuclear imaging technique used for diagnosing MI is perfusion scintigraphy or cold-spot imaging. Areas of the heart with normal perfusion and function have been shown to take up radioactive potassium and rubidium, permitting imaging of normal myocardium.[111,112] Defects in the normal pattern, known as cold-spots, represent areas of decreased flow or function, possibly associated with ischemia and acute or old myocardial infarction. The cold-spot technique is as highly sensitive for detection of MI (greater than 90%) as technetium-pyrophosphate hot-spot imaging, but is not as specific. Because of the high photon energies associated with radioactive potassium and rubidium, thallium-201 is now used for myocardial perfusion scintigraphy. After intravenous injection into a peripheral vein, this potassium analog is extracted by normal myocardium (85% extraction), providing images within minutes.

When flow is low to normal, thallium-201 is distributed within the myocardium in proportion to the regional myocardial blood flow. At higher flow rates, uptake is no longer linear, and substantial stress is required to achieve adequate imaging. Thallium-201 uptake also is related to myocardial function and levels of adenosine triphosphatase. With normal flow and function, the thallium image appears doughnut shaped. The central zone of decreased uptake reflects the ventricular cavity. All walls normally demonstrate activity; however, in approximately 20% of normal patients, the apical views will demonstrate a perfusion defect, despite normal function and flow in this area. Changes in coronary flow or function during ischemia or infarction reveal the areas of decreased perfusion, or cold-spots (Fig. 1-7).

Thallium-201 imaging is highly specific if performed within 6 hours of an acute MI.[113] This specificity decreases dramatically, how-

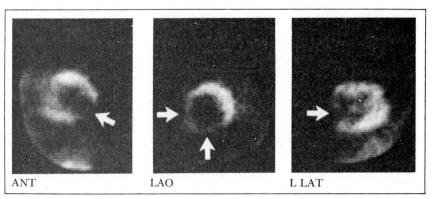

ANT   LAO   L LAT

FIGURE 1-7.   Resting thallium-201 myocardial perfusion scintigraphy shown in the anterior *(ANT)*, left anterior oblique *(LAO)*, and left lateral *(L LAT)* positions in a patient with a recent transmural myocardial infarction. Perfusion defects, as seen in the apical *(ANT)*, inferior and septal *(LAO)* regions. *(Cohn PF: Diagnosis and Therapy of Coronary Artery Disease. Boston, Little, Brown & Co, 1979)*

ever, approximately 24 hours after infarction, particularly in cases involving less than 5 grams of infarcted tissue. A comparison of hot-spot and cold-spot imaging is shown in Table 1-1.

Myocardial Perfusion Imaging.   Myocardial perfusion imaging using thallium-201 provides information about the extent, localization, reversibility and stress response of the coronary circulation, as well as a method for quantifying the functional significance of CAD. Quantifying the dysfunction associated with myocardial ischemia requires visible changes in thallium-201 uptake that depend on significant increases in coronary blood flow. In the absence of MI, however, coronary blood flow is relatively homogeneous throughout the ventricle, even with stenoses of up to 75%. In the resting state, perfusion defects cannot be detected unless coronary stenosis is severe (greater than 90%). Since stenotic vessels have limited coronary vascular reserve in response to metabolic stress, the normal resting homogeneous pattern of coronary perfusion can be disturbed and made heterogeneous during metabolic stress. Injection of the isotope during maximal stress then permits visualization of perfusion heterogeneities reflecting areas of ischemia. Because of the rapid myocardial clearance rate of thallium-201, redistribution of thallium occurs quickly, also allowing visualization of the reperfusion process.

Imaging is performed within 5 to 10 minutes of injection of thalli-

TABLE 1-1.   Hot-Spot Versus Cold-Spot Radionuclear Imaging

	Hot-Spot Imaging	Cold-Spot Imaging
Radionuclide	Technetium-99m pyrophosphate	Thallium-201
Uptake by	Infarcted tissue	Normal tissue (normal perfusion and metabolism)
Positive with	Acute MI (5 gm infarct)	Acute MI (5 gm infarct) Old MI Ischemia
Timing		
Earliest positive test	12–16 hours (post MI)	Immediately
Most sensitive	48–72 hours	24 hr
Other uses	Right ventricular MI Subendocardial MI Infarct size (+)	Chamber size LVH, RVH, ASH Stress testing

LVH = left ventricular hypertrophy; *RVH* = right ventricular hypertrophy; *ASH* = asymmetric septal hypertrophy

um-201 during maximal exercise or during infusion of a coronary vasodilator like dipyridamole, which produces effects simulating exercise. Perfusion defects, or cold-spots, are invisible for approximately 30 to 60 minutes, and redistribution usually occurs during the next 2 to 3 hours. Repeat imaging is performed approximately 3 to 4 hours after the first test to determine whether the initial perfusion defects persist or disappear. Those that persist indicate areas of infarction or prolonged ischemia (unlikely); those that disappear indicate areas of reversible perfusion defect or transient myocardial ischemia without infarction (Fig. 1-8).

The perfusion defect also may worsen, which is consistent with previous infarction with superimposed new myocardial ischemia. The highest sensitivities reported with this technique are 90%,[114–116] and the lowest are 60%, in patients with single-vessel disease involving the circumflex or right coronary arteries. Specificities are greater than 90%, with few false positives noted.

Dipyridamole thallium scintigraphy is useful in predicting outcome events in patients undergoing vascular surgery procedures,[15] particularly patients with marked peripheral vascular disease who are incapable of maximal or submaximal exercise. Although this technique has prognostic value, the costs and morbidity associated with it require further study to justify its use in a large patient population.

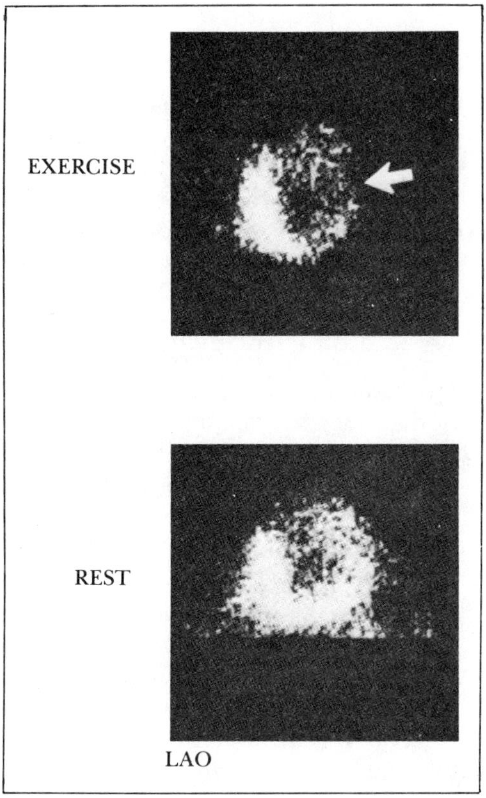

FIGURE 1-8. Exercise and resting thallium-201 myocardial perfusion scintigrams in the left anterior oblique *(LAO)* position in a patient with a reversible diffusion defect. During exercise, a lateral wall perfusion defect is noted *(arrow)*, which resolves with rest. This is consistent with transient myocardial ischemia. *(Cohn PF: Diagnosis and Therapy of Coronary Artery Disease. Boston, Little, Brown & Co, 1979)*

Tomography. The advantage of tomography over the previously described scintigraphic techniques is that it enables differentiation of different regions of the myocardium and isolation of background noise. Of the two forms of tomography available, limited-angle and transaxial-computed, only the latter appears to offer a significant advantage. With transaxial-computed tomography, the gamma camera is rotated through 180 or 360 degrees about the patient, making 32 or 64 stops at 20- to 40-second intervals. These data are processed, averaged, and summed, and images in multiple planes are produced. The LV appears horseshoe-shaped in a normal patient, with the open end of the horseshoe corresponding to the region of the aortic valve. Distribution of thallium-201 is homogeneous throughout the septum, including the anterior and lateral walls. As with thallium scintigraphy, the central perfusion defect represents the ventricular cavity.

Perfusion defects are more easily detected using tomography, because the images of the normally perfused and hypoperfused myocardium do not overlap as they do during thallium perfusion scintigraphy. Tomography enhances differentiation of myocardial tissue from other tissues, such as the lung. It also appears to have significant potential for precise definition of infarct size or degree of perfusion defect. It already is used to verify ambulatory ECG changes in studies of silent myocardial ischemia and promises to become the standard for verification of other clinical measures of ischemia.

Radionuclear Evaluation of Cardiac Mechanics

Two radionuclear techniques are presently available for evaluation of cardiac mechanics: first-pass radionuclide angiography and gated blood-pool imaging. Both provide ventricular function information, including ejection fraction, end-systolic and end-diastolic volumes, cardiac output, pulmonary transit time, and intracardiac shunt. The two techniques have distinct advantages.

First-pass Radionuclear Angiography. First-pass radionuclear angiography allows a temporal separation of the right and left sides of the heart, as well as the lung. With this technique, a bolus of radiopharmaceutical, usually technetium-99m, is injected into a peripheral or central vein, and radioactivity is counted as this bolus passes through the central circulation. The entire sequence is measured over 10 to 15 seconds and allows acute assessment of cardiac performance, particularly in unstable patients. Assessments should be made at multiple time intervals thereafter and require repeated injections of the radiopharmaceutical.

The scintillation counters usually are multicrystal and digital cameras allowing the required rapid acquisition and measurement of high radioisotope count. Ejection fraction, cardiac output, end-diastolic volume, pulmonary transit time, and shunt flow can be calculated using this technique.

A representative time–activity curve showing the transit of the radioisotope through the right and left ventricles is presented in Figure 1-9. Only the initial transit of the radioisotope is measured, which allows anatomic separation of the right and left ventricles. With each cardiac cycle, the measured activities at end-diastole and end-systole are proportional to the respective ventricular volumes. The maximum and minimum count rates during a cycle correspond to end-diastole and end-systole, respectively. Ejection fraction can be computed by the difference between the end-diastolic and end-systolic count rates,

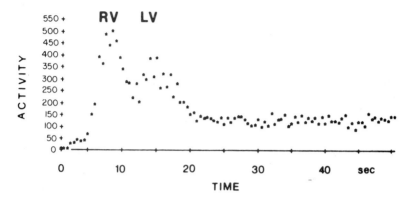

FIGURE 1-9. A normal time–activity curve demonstrating the first transit of the radiotracer through the right ventricle *(RV)* and the left ventricle *(LV)*. *(Ashburn WL et al: Left ventricular ejection fraction: A review of several radionuclide angiographic approaches using the scintillation camera. Progr Cardiovasc Dis 20:267, 1978)*

divided by the end-diastolic count, or subtracted from the background count. Typically, the ejection fraction is computed over three to five cycles and averaged. This first-pass ejection fraction technique correlates well with contrast angiography (r = 0.94 to 0.97).[117–119]

Right ventricular ejection fraction has been measured similarly. The variable and complex geometry of the right ventricle limits the precision of other techniques using geometric calculations. Using the first-pass technique, right ventricular ejection fraction has a mean normal value of 0.55, with a lower normal limit of 0.45.[120] Values have been determined for several clinical disorders, including congenital disease,[121,122] chronic obstructive pulmonary disease,[120,121] cystic fibrosis, and during MI.[123,124]

The first-pass technique can also be used for calculation of end-diastolic volume,[102] LV ejection phase indices such as ejection rate,[118] and peak diastolic filling rate.[125] These indices are difficult to validate, however, and only measurement of relative changes appears to be useful.

Gated Blood-Pool Imaging. The second radionuclide imaging technique used to evaluate ventricular performance is gated blood-pool imaging. Unlike the first-pass technique, the radionuclide is used to label blood products that remain within the intravascular space and create an equilibrium state. Radiopharmaceuticals, such as technetium 99-labeled human serum albumin or technetium 99-labeled red blood cells, are presently used. After the radionuclide equilibrates in the intravascular space, the gamma camera accumulates activity over the region of interest and identifies end-systole and end-diastole by gating to a physiologic marker, usually the R wave of the ECG. Data from 300 to 500 cardiac cycles are averaged to produce count rates of approximately 300,000 over the 2- to 10-minute imaging time, which cause a high resolution radionuclide angiocardiogram. Background activity is measured by selecting a noncardiac area (lung) and subtracting that activity from the measured cardiac volumes to produce a relative ventricular volume. As with the first-pass technique, ejection fraction is computed as the ratio of the difference between end-diastolic and end-systolic volume to the end-diastolic volume.

Regional ejection fraction and wall motion may be measured using a series of geometrical models and processing algorithms.[126-128] Absolute determinations are difficult to corroborate, but relative changes in these indices provide useful information. Valvular regurgitation can be calculated using the ratio of the right-to-left ventricular stroke counts as an index. Although the presence of regurgitation is detectable, quantifying it is difficult.[129]

Both first-pass and gated-pool radionuclide imaging provide accurate assessment of global LV ejection fraction, and the correlation between these methods is high (r = 0.87–0.89).[130,131] There are several important differences between these techniques, however, which are summarized in Table 1-2. Gated wall imaging is particularly useful when higher count rates are required, for example, to estimate regional wall motion. In studies where background plays a significant role, such as in edge detection, first-pass studies using lesser activity are more accurate. For monitoring clinical function over a period of up to 4 hours, gated wall imaging is superior. For interventional studies requiring multiple measurements, first-pass techniques are more suitable, although accumulation of background activity with each bolus injection limits the number of repeated studies possible.

Conclusions. Radionuclear imaging provides unique information for detection of MI, quantification of myocardial perfusion abnormalities, and calculation of ventricular performance and wall-motion indices. Knowledge of the techniques and ability to interpret the results are important to anesthesiologists seeking to enhance the preoperative assessment of MI and to quantify ventricular function.

TABLE 1-2.   First-pass Versus Gated-pool Radionuclear Angiography

	First-Pass	Gated-Pool
Radionuclide	Any technetium 99m-labeled pharmaceutical	Technetium (99m)-labeled albumin or RBC
Type of technique	Transient (30 secs) Multiple injections/hr	Steady state (6 hr) Single injection/hr
EF correlation with angiography	>0.90	>0.90
Uses	LVEF Exercise testing Dyskinesis RVEF Intracardiac shunt	LVEF Exercise testing Dyskinesis
Geometric assumptions	None	Several

EF = ejections fraction; *LVEF* = left ventricular ejection fraction; *RVEF* = right ventricular ejection fraction

Decisions regarding preoperative preparation, intraoperative and postoperative monitoring, and choice of therapeutics and anesthetic agents can benefit from their application.

Cardiac Catheterization

Cardiac catheterization is first credited to Claude Bernard (1844), who catheterized the left and right ventricles of a horse using a retrograde approach from the jugular vein and the carotid artery. The most significant developments of this technique are summarized in Table 1-3.

Indications.   The indications for cardiac catheterization and coronary arteriography vary widely. In patients in whom chest pain is the predominant symptom, cardiac catheterization is performed when angina is unstable, medically refractory, atypical (Prinzmetal's

TABLE 1-3.   History of Cardiac Catheterization

1844	Bernard: First catheterization of the right and left ventricles (horse).
1929	Forssmann: First catheterization of the right ventricle in humans.
1930	Kline: Catheterization of the right ventricle in 11 patients with measurement of cardiac output using the Fick technique.
1941	Cournand and Richards: Studies on right heart physiology in humans.
1947	Dexter: Studies of congenital heart disease, and first use of the pulmonary artery wedge position to obtain pulmonary capillary bed measurements.
1949	Dexter, Lagerlof & Werko: First measurement of pulmonary artery wedge pressures.
1950	Zimmerman & Larson: Retrograde left heart catheterization.
1953	Seldinger: Percutaneous technique for catheterization of the left and right heart chambers.
1959	Ross: Transseptal left heart catheterization.
1959	Sones: Selected coronary arteriography.
1970	Swan & Ganz: Introduction of the balloon-tipped, glove-guarded catheter.
1977	Gruentzig: Transluminal coronary angioplasty.

angina), or recurrent following cardiac surgery. In the absence of chest pain, cardiac catheterization is performed in patients with pump failure (usually after infarction), to evaluate valvular or congenital heart disease, or to evaluate coronary circulation after coronary artery bypass graft surgery.

Complications. A study of the morbidity and mortality associated with cardiac catheterization and arteriography in 89,079 patients, indicates an overall rate of 0.14%. In order of decreasing incidence, the morbid outcomes were contrast reaction (1.08%), ventricular fibrillation (0.76%), thrombosis (0.67%), MI (0.18%), hemorrhage (0.09%), cerebral embolus (0.09%), and pseudoaneurysm (0.04%). The only significant difference between the brachial and femoral approaches was the incidence of thrombosis, being 1.13% with the brachial approach, versus 0.20% with the femoral approach.

Techniques. The patient undergoing cardiac catheterization usually is fasting and premedicated with heparin (5000 units i.v.). In sequence, hemodynamic measurements, ventriculography, and coronary arteriography are performed.

Hemodynamic Measurements

In order to obtain hemodynamic measurements, a catheter is advanced into the aorta and LV, passing through the brachial or femoral artery. Coronary arteriography is performed using multiple views. For the left coronary artery the routine views are the left anterior oblique, anteroposterior, and right anterior oblique regions. The left lateral projection is occasionally used for further visualization of the left anterior descending coronary artery. To separate the proximal portions of the left circumflex and left anterior descending arteries, hemiaxial views are obtained with a left anterior oblique rotation and cranial–caudal angulation. The right coronary artery is visualized using right anterior oblique and left anterior oblique views.

The most commonly used contrast agent for arteriography and ventriculography is meglumine diatrizoate, the use of which has significantly decreased the incidence of ventricular fibrillation and asystole. Contrast reactions occur in approximately 1% of patients, however, resulting in hypotension, bradycardia, and T-wave changes on the ECG. Injections into the right coronary artery characteristically produce T-wave inversions in lead II, while left coronary-artery injection produces T-wave peaking. Approximately 10 to 20 ml of contrast agent is necessary to visualize the coronary arteries; two thirds of this amount is needed to visualize the left coronary arteries.

After injection of contrast agent, a series of hemodynamic measurements and calculations are made, including: systemic, pulmonary, and intracardiac pressure measurements; calculations of cardiac output, vascular resistance, oxygen consumption, and arteriovenous oxygen difference; and valve areas. Measurements of the right heart usually are also performed, by placing a catheter in the brachial or femoral vein. Normal values for these hemodynamic measurements are shown in Tables 1-4 and 1-5.

Cardiac Output. Cardiac output can be calculated using the Fick oxygen-method technique, the indicator-dilution technique, or ventriculography measurements. Pulmonary blood flow can be calculated by measuring oxygen consumption and the arteriovenous oxygen difference across the lungs. The following formula is used:

$$\text{Cardiac index (1/min/m}^2) = \frac{O_2 \text{ consumption (ml/min/m}^2)}{\text{arteriovenous } O_2 \text{ difference (ml/1)}}$$

TABLE 1-4.   Intracardiac and Pulmonary Pressure Measurements

	Pressure (mm Hg)		
	Systolic	*Diastolic*	*Mean*
Right atrium	—	—	−2–6
Right ventricle	15–30	0–8	5–15
Pulmonary artery	15–30	0–12	5–18
Pulmonary wedge	—	—	0–12
Left atrium	—	—	0–12
Left ventricle	100–140	60–90	70–105

TABLE 1-5.   Other Cardiovascular Measurements

Left ventricle	
End-diastolic	70–95
End-systolic	24–36
Performance	
Cardiac output	2.5–4.2L/min/m^2
Stroke volume index	50–70 ml/m^2
Ejection fraction	0.67 ± 0.08 (SD)
Resistance (dynes/sec/cm^{-5})	
Pulmonary vascular	20–120
Systemic vascular	770–1500
Oxygen Measurements	
Oxygen consumption	110–150 ml/min/m^2
Arteriovenous oxygen difference	3–5 ml/100 ml blood
Valve Measurements (cm^4)	
Aortic valve area	2.6–3.5
Mitral valve area	4.0–6.0

Oxygen Consumption and Saturation. Oxygen consumption is measured by collecting expired air over a 3-minute period. The oxygen content is calculated from the ratio of the partial pressure of oxygen to the corrected barometric pressure, then from the product of the expired air oxygen consumption and minute ventilation. Arteriovenous oxygen difference is calculated from the oxygen content. The time-consuming technique of Van Slyke and Neill[132] has generally been replaced by reflectance oximetry for the measurement of oxygen saturation. Oxygen content can then be calculated from the product of hemoglobin concentration and saturation.

The indicator-dilution method is similar to the Fick method, but uses indocyanine green dye as an indicator. The dye is rapidly injected as a bolus into the pulmonary artery, and dye concentration is recorded from a systemic artery (brachial, femoral, or radial). The cardiac output is calculated from the arterial concentration curve (concentration versus time) using the equation:

$$\text{Cardiac output} = V_i/(C \times T)$$

where V_i is the volume of dye injected, C is the average concentration of the indicator during its first pass, and T is the total duration of the curve. C and T may be calculated from the curve by using planimetry or, more conveniently, electronic signal-processing techniques. The Fick method is analogous to this, but uses oxygen as the dye. When cardiac output is normal or elevated, the values obtained using the indicator-dilution and the Fick methods agree. When cardiac outputs are low, or when valvular regurgitation or intracardiac shunt exists, the indicator-dilution method becomes inaccurate.

The third and most commonly used method of computing cardiac output is ventriculography. By quantifying the end-diastolic and end-systolic images, ventricular volumes can be approximated. The difference between the end-diastolic and end-systolic volumes, or the stroke volume, multiplied by the heart rate, equals the cardiac output. This method, although less accurate than the Fick method, yields acceptable cardiac output measurements, except when aortic or mitral regurgitation or atrial fibrillation is present.

Vascular Resistance. Systemic vascular resistance and pulmonary vascular resistance (SVR, PVR) are calculated from the measurements of these pressures and cardiac output, using the formulae:

$$\text{SVR (dynes} \cdot \text{sec} \cdot \text{cm}^{-5}) = \frac{80 \times (\text{BP–RA})}{\dot{Q}_s}$$

$$\text{PVR (dynes} \cdot \text{sec} \cdot \text{cm}^{-5}) = \frac{80 \times (\text{PA–LA})}{\dot{Q}_p}$$

where BP, RA, PA, LA are the mean aortic, right atrial, pulmonary arteries, and the left atrial blood pressures, respectively, in mmHg. $\dot{Q}s$ and $\dot{Q}_p$ are the systemic and pulmonary blood flows in L/min. The normal ranges for resistance are shown in Table 1-4.

Shunt. Intracardiac shunts are calculated from pulmonary and systemic blood flows using the Fick principle. Pulmonary blood flow is defined as:

$$\dot{Q}_p \text{ (min)} = \frac{O_2 \text{ consumption (ml/min)}}{\text{PVO}_2 \text{ content - PA O}_2 \text{ content (ml/min)}}$$

where PV and PA are the pulmonary venous and pulmonary arterial values.
Systemic blood flow is defined as:

$$\dot{Q}_s \text{ (min)} = \frac{O_2 \text{ consumption (ml/min)}}{\text{A O}_2 \text{ content–PA O}_2 \text{ content (ml/min)}}$$

where A refers to the arterial blood. With a left-to-right shunt (atrial septal defect, ventricular septal defect, patent ductus arteriosus), pulmonary blood flow is greater than systemic blood flow, and pulmonary oxygen saturation is greater than mixed-venous saturation. Shunts can be localized anatomically from the oxygen saturation measurements sampled in the cardiac chambers. This technique is sensitive, except for small shunts, ($\dot{Q}_p/\dot{Q}_s \leq 1.3$). These may be detected from hydrogen gas measurements, using a right heart hydrogen-sensitive electrode to measure direct current voltage changes. Right-to-left shunts can be detected clinically and may be detected from relative desaturations. Small right-to-left shunts can be detected using indocyanine dye injections.

Valve Area. The orifice area of the aortic and mitral valves is calculated from the flow through the valve and the pressure gradient across it,[133–135] using the following formulae:

$$\text{Aortic valve area (cm}^2\text{)} = \frac{F}{44.5 \times \sqrt{\Delta P}}$$

$$\text{Mitral valve area (cm}^2\text{)} = \frac{F}{38 \times \sqrt{\Delta P}}$$

where F is the flow through the orifice in ml/sec, and P is the mean pressure gradient across the orifice in mmHg (see Table 1-4). The constants 44.5 and 38 incorporate the effects of the viscous resistance to flow and turbulent flow. The flow through the valve is calculated from:

$$\text{Flow (ml/sec)} = \frac{\text{Cardiac output (ml/min)}}{\text{DFP (sec/min) or SEP (sec/min)}}$$

where DFP is the diastolic filling period and SEP is the systolic ejection period.

Regurgitant Fraction. The aortic or mitral valve regurgitant fraction can be calculated from the ventriculographic stroke volume and the Fick stroke volume. The ventriculographic stroke volume, derived from the difference between the end-diastolic and end-systolic volumes, represents the total stroke volume, or the combination of the forward and regurgitant volumes. The Fick stroke volume represents the forward stroke volume. The difference between the ventriculographic volume and the Fick volume is the regurgitant stroke volume. The regurgitant fraction (RF) is defined as:

$$RF = \frac{\text{Ventriculographic SV–Fick SV}}{\text{Ventriculographic SV}}$$

Regurgitant fractions greater than 30% have been considered to be hemodynamically important.

Coronary Sinus Flow. Coronary sinus blood flow may be calculated using a thermodilution technique.[136] The thermodilution catheter is advanced into the coronary sinus from the right antecubital vein. Coronary sinus flow can be determined from temperature measurements of the injectate, the downstream blood, and the body by using standard formulae.[136] It also can be determined by injecting inert gas (xenon) into the coronary artery and recording the radioactivity washout with a scintillation camera. Regional myocardial blood flow can be derived from the radioactivity curve, the partition coefficient of the isotope in myocardial tissue, and the specific gravity of the myocardial tissue.

Ventriculography Measurements

Left ventriculography usually is performed after hemodynamic measurements are made, and before coronary arteriography is performed. With the catheter positioned beneath the mitral valve leaflets, a test injection of approximately 10 to 15 ml of contrast is given over a 1-second period. The ventriculogram is then obtained in either the 30° right anterior oblique projection alone or in combination with a 60° left anterior oblique projection. Approximately 35 ml of contrast material containing diatrizoate meglumine and diatrizoate sodium (Renografin-76[R]) is injected into the LV for 3 to 4 seconds. The diastolic and systolic phases of the ventricular cycle are recorded on 35mm cine film.

End-diastolic and end-systolic volume measurements can be made using the area-length method, based on formulae developed by Dodge.[137] Both single-plane and biplane volume determinations can be measured using the equation:

$$V = \frac{4}{3} \times \frac{L}{2} \times \frac{D_a}{2} \times \frac{D_b}{2}$$

where V is volume (ml), L is the major axis length (cm), and D_a and D_b are the minor axis lengths (cm) in the right or left anterior oblique projections. Modifications of this formula also are used.[137] Ventriculographic stroke volume can be calculated as the difference between the end-diastolic and the end-systolic volumes. Cardiac output is the product of stroke times heart rate, and ejection fraction is the ratio of stroke volume to end-diastolic volume. The normal values for these variables are shown in Table 1-4.

Ventriculography also is used to estimate the velocity of circumferential fiber shortening, the mean ejection rate and wall thickness, LV mass, and stress.[137,138]

Segmental wall motion abnormalities are visualized using ventriculography and may be quantified from ventriculography. Ventricular dyssynergy has several abnormal contraction patterns—hypokinesis, akinesis, dyskinesis, and hyperkinesis (Fig. 1-10). These

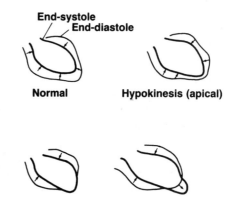

FIGURE 1-10. Segmental wall-motion abnormalities contrasting normal wall motion with apical hypokinesis, akinesis, and dyskinesis. *(Kaplan J (ed): Cardiac Anesthesia, 2nd ed, p 376. Orlando, FL, Grune & Stratton, 1987)*

abnormalities can be quantified using several techniques, including calculation of hemiaxial shortening, area ejection fraction, and the percentage of dyssynergic segments.[137,139] These methods superimpose the ventricular silhouettes at end-systole and end-diastole and can be applied manually or with computerized image processing systems.[140] An example of axis-shortening calculations is shown in Figure 1-11.

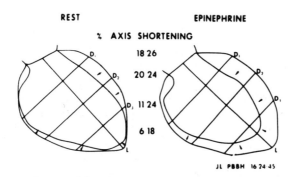

FIGURE 1-11. The change in axis shortening with administration of epinephrine is demonstrated. The percent axial shortening is shown for three minor axes *(D₁, D₂, and D₃)* and the long axis *(L)*. *(Horn HR et al: Augmentation of left contraction pattern in coronary artery disease by an inotropic catecholamine. The epinephrine ventriculogram. Circulation 49:1063, 1974)*

Biplane ventriculography is used to identify wall-motion abnormalities in patients who have previous MI, cardiomegaly, or
congestive heart failure. Intervention ventriculography (two-state
or dynamic ventriculography) is performed to determine latent
ventricular dysfunction, or contractile reserve. Latent ventricular
dysfunction is assessed by inducing myocardial ischemia using
atrial pacing, dynamic exercise, or static exercise. Myocardial ischemia introduces new segmental wall-motion abnormalities that
may cause decreased LV performance (depressed ejection fraction).
The hemodynamic significance of an obstructive coronary artery
lesion also can be assessed this way. The contractile reserve of
the LV can be estimated using inotropic stimulation (catecholamine
infusion, postextrasystolic potentiation) or by decreasing preload (nitroglycerin). With the first technique, an initial ventriculogram is obtained, epinephrine is infused, and a second ventriculogram is performed to compare wall-motion contractile patterns.
Postextrasystolic potentiation is obtained by inducing a premature
contraction by manipulation of the right heart catheter or by pacemaker R-wave triggering. Ventricular unloading is assessed using
0.4 mg of nitroglycerin sublingually to determine the reversibility
of dyssynergy.

Comparison of Measures of Myocardial Function. The relative
specificity and sensitivity of measures of myocardial function have
been studied in 317 patients with CAD, but not with valvular heart
disease.[141] The most specific indices, in order of decreasing specificity, were the ejection fraction, degree of dyssynergy, stroke work,
end-diastolic volume, end-systolic volume, cardiac index, and end-
diastolic pressure. The specificity was greater than 0.80 for all of these
indices except cardiac output (0.59–0.77) and end-diastolic pressure
(0.53–0.59), but sensitivity was low except for ventricular dyssynergy
(less than 0.50). From these data, it appears that ventricular dysfunction is best predicted by the ejection fraction and the degree of dyssynergy, with abnormalities of these variables commonly associated
with abnormalities in ventricular output (cardiac output, stroke
work), filling (end-diastolic volume and end-diastolic pressure), and
ejection (end-systolic volume). Abnormality of the stroke work index,
end-diastolic volume, and end-systolic volume appear to be good indicators of ventricular dysfunction. Cardiac output is a marginal index, associated with normality of the other indices 23% to 41% of the
time.

Coronary Arteriography

For coronary arteriography, a Sones catheter or a Judkins catheter is advanced into the heart. With the Sones technique, the catheter is advanced into the aorta by a right brachial arteriotomy; with the Judkins technique, the femoral artery is directly punctured using a Seldinger needle, and the catheter is then advanced into the aorta. The normal dimensions of the right coronary artery are 3.7 (± 1.1) mm by 2.4 (± 0.9) mm. The dimensions of the left coronary artery are 4.7 (± 1.2) mm by 3.2 (± 1.1) mm. Lesions involving less than 50% of the luminal diameter (approximately 75% of the cross-sectional area) usually are not hemodynamically significant. Those involving 75% or more of the luminal diameter are considered significant, although the accuracy of coronary-artery visualization has been questioned.[142]

The degree of stenosis can be estimated by comparing the vessel widths of the stenotic and prestenotic (normal) segments, using angled projections to enhance visualization of the coronary system. Various quantification and coding systems exist, along with computer-assisted programs.[143]

Coronary collaterals usually are not detected in normal hearts. Coronary arteries typically lie freely on the epicardial surface of the heart. Coronary anastomoses, when visualized, are either intercoronary or intersegmental. An intercoronary anastomosis usually involves two of the three principal coronary arteries, while the intersegmental anastomosis joins two points along the same artery.

Interventional Techniques

Coronary-artery spasm may be induced for diagnostic purposes using ergonovine maleate, as well as morphine, alpha and beta stimulants and blockers, cholinergic and anticholinergic agents, and calcium channel blockers. Spontaneous spasm and resolution of that spasm with the administration of sublingual nitrate was first described by Prinzmetal and colleagues.[24] Spasm also may occur with fixed coronary obstructions or may be iatrogenically produced by catheter manipulation.

Intracoronary thrombolysis was first induced by administration of fibrinolysin during acute MI.[144,145] Streptokinase was later introduced for use in thrombotic occlusion during the evolving stage of an acute MI. Rentrop[146] reported recanalization of occluded arteries in over 75% of patients during the acute stages of MI using this technique. Schwarz and coworkers[147] demonstrated that the success of this procedure is related to the duration of ischemia and suggested that early recognition and prompt treatment enhances the success.

Transluminal coronary angioplasty[148] appears to be most useful in patients with recent-onset angina and a single, proximal concentric stenosis of a major epicardial coronary artery. Higher risk subgroups now also undergo angioplasty, including patients with multivessel disease, distal stenoses, eccentric and calcified lesions, and previous coronary artery bypass graft surgery and evolving MI.[148–152] A typical technique involves pretreatment with nifedipine (20 mg sublingual) for coronary spasm, and advancement of the #8 French catheter into the coronary ostium. After a diagnostic angiogram, intracoronary nitroglycerin is injected. Anticoagulation is monitored throughout the procedure to prevent thrombotic complications. After insertion of a guiding catheter, a dilating catheter system is introduced. The inflated balloon diameter varies from 2 to 4 mm in diameter and is usually 25 mm in length. The initial inflations are performed for 10 to 20 seconds. Patients are monitored, and signs of chest pain or ST elevation are noted. Repeat inflations are performed with increasing pressures until hemodynamic and angiographic results occur. A gradient across the stenosis of 15 mm Hg or less is attempted.

In a study of 3,079 patients undergoing coronary angioplasty,[153] the success rate was 65%, the complication rate was 20%, and the mortality rate was 0.8%. The morbid outcomes included coronary dissection, occlusion, or spasm (10.4%), MI (5.5%), ventricular tachycardia (2.3%), and prolonged angina (6.7%). The mean age of the population was 54 years, with 26% of the patients in Canadian heart-class IV and 37% in Canadian heart-class III. Seventy-three percent of the patients had single-vessel disease, with 64% of these involving the left anterior descending artery. One year after angioplasty, 72% (1,397) of patients maintained successful results and did not require repeat angioplasty or coronary-artery bypass surgery; 12% required repeat dilation.

Magnetic Resonance Imaging and Spectroscopy

Magnetic resonance imaging, used to characterize molecular structures, has recently been shown to provide high-resolution tomographic and three-dimensional images of the heart. In addition, spectroscopic information can quantify metabolic derangements.

Although this method is costly, it is noninvasive and safe, since it does not require the use of ionizing radiation.

Certain nuclei with an odd number of protons and neutrons have an intrinsic net nuclear spin. The spinning charged nucleus generates a magnetic field that can be imaged. Photons, carbon-13, sodium-23, and phosphorus-31 nuclei exhibit such magnetic moments and are used for magnetic imaging. The concentration of these magnetic nuclei in a sample can be determined by placing the sample in an external magnetic field. Before placement in the magnetic field, the magnetic moments are randomly oriented. After placement, magnetic moments are aligned in the same or opposite direction as the field, resulting in a macroscopic magnetic moment, whose magnitude is related to the concentration of the magnetic nuclei (such as phosphorus-31) in the sample.

Unlike computed tomography, magnetic resonance imaging can be gated to the cardiac cycle, allowing assessment of LV function.[154] Ischemic insults to the heart may also be detectable because prolonged ischemia affects proton relaxation parameters. Increased signal intensities in ischemic regions appear to be associated with lipid accumulation, edema and fibrosis. Magnetic resonance imaging may also allow characterization of ischemia and quantification of its extent. Recent advances include a proton imaging technique, which allows acquisition of the entire image in less than 100 milliseconds,[155] and sodium-23 images, which characterize the blood pool in the isolated beating rat heart.[156] Turnover of high-energy phosphates can be quantified, and the accumulation of inorganic phosphorus in acutely ischemic tissue can be detected using phosphorus-31 spectroscopy.

Magnetic resonance imaging also may be used for metabolic assessment of ischemic segment function using high-energy phosphate turnover and intracellular pH calculations. It also may be used in combination with coronary angiography and myocardial perfusion imaging.

Summary

Perioperative cardiac morbidity remains a significant problem throughout the world. The accurate identification of at-risk patients will help to determine beneficial monitoring and therapeutic regimens throughout the perioperative period. The evaluation of patients with cardiac disease poses particular challenges, however. First, patients can present with a myriad of symptom complexes having varying degrees of clinical and subclinical ventricular dysfunction. Secondly, this age of cost-containment increases pressure to expedite the preoperative assessment of come-and-go and come-and-stay surgical patients, despite the increasing number and cost of preoperative cardiac tests. Consequently, anesthesiologists must have a thorough understanding of the types of preoperative cardiac tests available, the information they provide, and the indications for their use. We hope to have provided a source of information for the routine and nonroutine preoperative tests now available.

References

1. Mangano DT: Perioperative cardiac morbidity. Anesthesiology 72:153, 1990
2. Knapp RB, Topkins MJ, Artusio JF: The cerebrovascular accident and coronary occlusion in anesthesia. JAMA 182:322, 1962
3. Topkins MJ, Artusio JF: Myocardial infarction and surgery: A five year study. Anesth Analg 43:716, 1964
4. Tarhan S, Moffitt E, Taylor WF et al: Myocardial infarction after general anesthesia. JAMA 220:1451, 1972
5. Goldman L: Supraventricular tachyarrhythmias in hospitalized adults after surgery. Chest 73:450, 1978
6. Steen PA, Tinker JH, Tarhan S: Myocardial reinfarction after anesthesia and surgery. JAMA 239:2566, 1978
7. Rao TK, Jacobs KH, El-Etr AA: Reinfarction following anesthesia in patients with myocardial infarction. Anesthesiology 59:499, 1983
8. Hicks GL, Eastland MW, DeWeese JA et al: Survival improvement following aortic aneurysm resection. Ann Surg 181:863, 1975
9. Young AE, Sandberg GW, Couch NP: The reduction of mortality of abdominal aortic aneurysm resection. Am J Surg 134:585, 1977
10. Cooperman M, Pflug B, Martin EW Jr et al: Cardiovascular risk factors in patients with peripheral vascular disease. Surgery 84:505, 1978
11. Riles TS, Kopelman I, Imparato AM: Myocardial infarction following carotid endarterectomy: A review of 683 operations. Surgery 85:249, 1979
12. Hertzer NR: Fatal myocardial infarction following lower extremity revascularization. Two hundred seventy-three patients followed six to eleven postoperative years. Ann Surg 193:4, 1981
13. Hertzer NR: Myocardial ischemia. Surgery 93:97, 1983
14. Cutler BS, Wheeler HB, Paraskos JA et al: Applicability and interpretation of electrocardiographic stress testing in patients with peripheral vascular disease. Am J Surg 141:501, 1981
15. Boucher CA, Brewster DC, Darling CR et al: Determination of cardiac risk by dipyridamole-thallium imaging before peripheral vascular surgery. N Engl J Med 312:389, 1985

16. Kaplan JA, King SB: The precordial electrocardiographic lead (V5) in patients who have coronary artery disease. Anesthesiology 45:570, 1976
17. Kotrly KJ, Kotter GS, Mortara D et al: Intraoperative detection of myocardial ischemia with an ST segment trend monitoring system. Anesth Analg 63:343, 1984
18. Slogoff S, Keats AS: Does perioperative myocardial ischemia lead to postoperative myocardial infarction? Anesthesiology 62:107, 1985
19. Schluter M, Hinrichs A, Thier W et al: Transesophageal two-dimensional echocardiography: Comparison of ultrasonic and anatomic sections. Am J Cardiol 53:1173, 1984
20. Coriat P, Daloz M, Bousseau D et al: Prevention of intraoperative myocardial ischemia during noncardiac surgery with intravenous nitroglycerin. Anesthesiology 61:193, 1984
21. Diamond GA, Forrester JS: Analysis of probability as an aid in the clinical diagnosis of coronary-artery disease. N Engl J Med 1350, 1979
22. Mangano DT, Hedgcock M, Wisneski JA. Predictive value of the chest radiograph in patients with coronary artery disease. Anesthesiology (in press)
23. CASS: Coronary Artery Surgery Study (CASS): Manual of Operations II: Data Collection and Storage. Collaborative Studies in Coronary Artery Surgery. Washington, D.C.: National Heart, Lung and Blood Institute, prepared by the CASS Coordinating Center,
24. Prinzmetal M, Kennamer R, Merliss R et al: A variant form of angina pectoris. Am J Med 27:375, 1959
25. Cohn PF: Silent myocardial ischemia as a manifestation of asymptomatic coronary artery disease: What is appropriate therapy? Am J Cardiol 56:28D, 1985
26. Deanfield JE, Selwyn AP, Chierchia S et al: Myocardial ischemia during daily life in patients with stable angina: Its relation to symptoms and heart rate changes. Lancet ii:753, 1983
27. Deanfield JE, Ribiero P, Oakley K et al: Analysis of ST segment changes in normal subjects: Implication for ambulatory monitoring in angina pectoris. Am J Cardiol 54:1321, 1984
28. Herrick JB: Clinical features of sudden obstruction of the coronary arteries. JAMA 59:2015, 1912
29. Gorham LW, Martin SJ: Coronary artery occlusion with and without pain. Arch Intern Med 112:821, 1938
30. Stroud WD, Wagner JA: Silent or atypical coronary occlusion. Ann Intern Med 15:25-32, 1941
31. Cohn PF: Severe asymptomatic coronary artery disease: A diagnostic, prognostic and therapeutic puzzle. Am J Med 62:565, 1977
32. Deanfield JE, Shea M, Ribiero P et al: Transient ST-segment depression as a marker of myocardial ischemia during daily life. Am J Cardiol 54:1195, 1984
33. Kennedy JA: The incidence of myocardial infarction without pain in autopsied cases. Am Heart J 14:703, 1937
34. Boyd LD, Werblow SC: Coronary thrombosis without pain. Am J Med Sci 194:814, 1937

35. Johnson WJ, Achor RWP, Burchell HB: Unrecognized myocardial infarction. Arch Intern

36. Gordon T, Moore FE, Shurtleff D: Some methodologic problems in the long-term study of cardiovascular disease: Observation on the Framingham Study. J Chronic Dis 10:186, 1959

37. Lindberg HA, Berkson DM, Stamler J: Totally asymptomatic myocardial infarction: An estimate of its incidence in the living population. Arch Intern Med 106:628, 1960

38. Friedman GD, Kannel WB, Dawber TR: An evaluation of follow-up methods in the Framingham Heart Study. Am J Public Health 57:1015, 1967

39. Cohn PF, Gorlin R, Cohn LH et al: Left ventricular ejection fraction as a prognostic guide in surgical treatment of coronary and valvular heart disease. Am J Cardiol 34:136, 1979

40. Mangano DT: Biventricular function after myocardial revascularization in humans: Deterioration and recovery patterns during the first 24 hours. Anesthesiology 62:571, 1985

40a. Braunwald E, Ross J Jr, Sonnenblick ES: Mechanism of Contraction of the Normal and Failing Heart, 2nd ed, pp 166–200. Boston, Little Brown and Co, 1976

41. Mangano DT, Hedgcock MD, Wisneski J: Non-invasive prediction of ventricular dysfunction: Valvular heart disease. Anesthesiology 63:3A, 1985

42. Cohn PF, Vokonas PS, Williams RA et al: Diastolic heart sounds and filling waves in coronary artery disease. Circulation 44:196, 1971

43. Cohn PF, Thompson P, Strauss W: Diastolic heart sounds during static (handgrip) exercise in patients with chest pain. Circulation 47:1217, 1973

44. Fischl S, Gorlin R, Herman MV: The intermediate coronary syndrome: Clinical, angiographic and therapeutic aspects. N Engl J Med 288:1193, 1973

45. Martin CE, Shaver JA, Leonard JJ et al: Physical signs, apexcardiography, phonocardiography and systolic time intervals in angina pectoris. Circulation 46:1098, 1972

46. Spodick DH, Quarry VM: Prevalence of the fourth heart sound by phonocardiography in the absence of cardiac disease. Am Heart J 87:11, 1974

47. Goldman L, Caldera DL, Nussbaum SR et al: Multifactorial index of cardiac risk in noncardiac surgical procedures. N Engl J Med 297:845, 1977

48. Cohn PF, Gabbay SI, Weglicki WB: Serum lipid levels in angiographically-defined coronary artery disease. Ann Intern Med 84:241, 1976

49. Gotto AM, Gorry GA, Thompson JR et al: Relationship between plasma lipid concentration and coronary artery disease in 496 patients. Circulation 56:875, 1977

50. Marcella JJ, Nichols AB, Johnson LL et al: Exercise-induced myocardial ischemia in patients with coronary artery disease: Lack of evidence for platelet activation or fibrin formation in peripheral venous blood. J Am Coll Cardiol 1:1185, 1983

51. Shell WE, Kjekshus JK, Sobel BE: Quantitative assessment of the extent

of myocardial infarction in the conscious dog by means of analysis of serial changes in serum creatine phosphokinase activity. J Clin Invest 50:2614, 1971

52. Sobel BE, Shell WE: Serum enzyme determination in the diagnosis and assessment of myocardial infarction. Circulation 45:471, 1972

53. Grande P, Hansen BF, Christiansen C: Estimation of acute myocardial infarct size in man by serum CK-MB measurements. Circulation 65:756, 1982

54. Weidner N: Laboratory diagnosis of acute myocardial infarct. Usefulness of determination of lactate dehydrogenase (LDH)-1 level and the ratio of LDH-1 to total LDH. Arch Pathol Lab Med 106:375, 1982

55. Gorlin R: Coronary Artery Disease, p 177. Philadelphia, WB Saunders, 1976

56. Dressler W, Roesler H: High T waves in the earliest stage of myocardial infarction. Am Heart J 34:627, 1947

57. Madias JE: The earliest electrocardiographic sign of acute transmural myocardial infarction. J Electrocardiol 10:193, 1977

58. Pardee HEB: An electrocardiographic sign of coronary artery obstruction. Arch Intern Med 26:244, 1920

59. Abbott JA, Scheinman MM: Nondiagnostic electrocardiogram in patients with acute myocardial infarction: Clinical and anatomic correlations. Am J Med 55:608, 1973

60. Autenrieth G, Surawicz B, Kuo CS et al: Primary T wave abnormalities caused by uniform and regional shortening of ventricular monophasic action potential in dog. Circulation 51:668, 1975

61. Bartel AG, Chen JT, Peter RH et al: The significance of coronary calcification detected by fluoroscopy. A report of 360 patients. Circulation 49:1247, 1974

62. Hamby RI, Tabrah F, Wisoff BG et al: Coronary artery calcification: Clinical implications and angiographic correlates. Am Heart J 87:565, 1974

63. Einthoven W: Weiteres uber das elektrokardiogramm. Arch Fuer Gesamte Physiologie des Menschen und der Tiere 172:517, 1908

64. Feil H, Siegel ML: Electrocardiographic changes during attacks of angina pectoris. Am J Med Sci 175:255, 1928

65. Master AM, Oppenheimer ET: A simple exercise tolerance test for circulatory efficiency with standard tables for normal individuals. Am J Med Sci 177:223, 1929

66. Goldhammer S, Scherf D: Elektrokardiographische Untersuchungen Bei Kranker mit Angina Pectoris ("Ambulatorischer Typus") Zschr Klin Med 122:134, 1933

67. Rochmis P, Blackburn H: Exercise tests. A survey of procedures, safety and litigation experience in approximately 170,000 tests. JAMA 217:1061, 1971

68. Bruce RA, DeRouen TA, Blake B: Maximal exercise predictors of coronary heart disease events among asymptomatic men in Seattle Heart Watch. Circulation 56 (Suppl 3):15, 1977

69. Ellestad MH: Stress Testing: Principles and Practice. Philadelphia, FA Davis, 1975

70. Astrand P, Rodahl K: Evaluation of physical work capacity on the basis

of tests. In Van Dalen DB (ed): Textbook of Work Physiology: Physiological Bases of Exercise, 2nd ed. New York, McGraw-Hill, 1977

71. Sheffield LT: Exercise stress testing. In Braunwald E (ed): Heart Disease: A Textbook of Cardiovascular Medicine, p 267 Philadelphia, WB Saunders, 1984

72. Froelicher VF Jr, Yanowitz FG, Thompson AJ et al: The correlation of coronary angiography and the electrocardiographic response to maximal treadmill testing in 76 asymptomatic men. Circulation 48:597, 1973

73. Erikssen J, Rasmussen K, Forfany K et al: Exercise ECG and case history in the diagnosis of latent coronary heart disease among presumably healthy middle-aged men. Eur J Cardiol 5:463, 1977

74. Goldman S, Tselos S, Cohn K: Marked depth of ST-segment depression during treadmill exercise testing: Indicator of severe coronary artery disease. Chest 69:729, 1976

75. Dagenais GR, Rouleau JR, Christen A et al: Survival of patients with a strongly positive exercise electrocardiogram. Circulation 65:452, 1982

76. Schneider RM, Seaworth JF, Dohrmann ML et al: Anatomic and prognostic implications of an early positive treadmill exercise test. Am J Cardiol 50:682, 1982

77. Weiner DA, McCabe CH, Ryan TJ: Prognostic assessment of patients with coronary artery disease by exercise testing. Am Heart J 105:749, 1983

78. Brody DA: A theoretical analysis of intracavitary blood mass influence on the heart–lead relationship. Circ Res 4:731, 1956

79. Bonoris P, Greenberg PS, Castellanet M et al: Significance of changes in R wave amplitude during treadmill testing: Angiographic correlation. Am J Cardiol 41:846, 1978

80. Bonoris PE, Greenberg PS, Christison GW et al: Evaluation of R wave amplitude changes versus ST-segment depression in stress testing. Circulation 57:904, 1978

81. Hollenberg M, Go M, Massie BM et al: Influence of R wave amplitude on exercise-induced ST depression: Need for a "gain factor" correction when interpreting stress electrocardiograms. Am J Cardiol 56:13, 1985

82. Morris SN, McHenry PL: Incidence and significance of decreases in systolic blood pressure during graded treadmill exercise testing. Am J Cardiol 41:221, 1978

83. Feigenbaum H: Echocardiography, 3rd ed. Philadelphia, Lea & Febiger, 1981

84. Helak JW, Plappert T, Muhammad A: Two dimensional echocardiographic imaging of the left ventricle: Comparison of mechanical and phased array systems in vitro. Am J Cardiol 48:728, 1981

85. Eaton LW, Maughan WL, Shoukas AA et al: Accurate volume determination in the isolated ejecting canine left ventricle by two-dimensional echocardiography. Circulation 60:4, 1979

86. Folland ED, Parisi AF, Moynihan PF: Assessment of left ventricular ejection fraction and volumes by real-time, two-dimensional echocardiography. Circulation 60:4, 1979

87. Rushmer RF, Baker DW, Stegal HF: Transcutaneous Doppler flow detection as a nondestructive technique. J Appl Physiol 21:554, 1966

88. Strandness DE, McCutcheon EP, Rushmer RF: Application of a transcutaneous Doppler flow meter in evaluation of occlusive arterial disease. Surg Gynecol Obstet 122:1039, 1966

89. Sigel B, Popley GL, Boland J et al: Augmentation of flow sounds in the ultrasonic detection of venous abnormalities. Invest Radiol 2:256, 1967

90. Lavenson GS, Rich NM, Baugh JH: Value of ultrasonic flow detection in the management of peripheral vascular disease. Am J Surg 120:522, 1970

91. Block PJ, Popp RL: Two-dimensional echocardiographic assessment of left main coronary artery disease in man (abstract). Circulation 68 (Suppl II): 1463, 1983

92. Rink LD, Feigenbaum H, Godley RW et al: Echocardiographic detection of left main coronary artery obstruction. Circulation 65:719, 1982

93. Friedman MJ, Sahn DJ, Goldman S et al: High predictive accuracy for detection of left main coronary artery disease by antilog signal processing of two-dimensional echocardiographic images. Am Heart J 103:194, 1982

94. Heger JJ, Weyman AE, Wann LS et al: Cross-sectional echocardiography in acute myocardial infarction: detection and localization of regional left ventricular asynergy. Circulation 60:531, 1979

95. Corya BC, Rasmussen S, Feigenbaum H, Knoebel S, Black MJ: Systolic thickening and thinning of the septum and posterior wall in patients with coronary artery disease, congestive cardiomyopathy and atrial sepal defect. Circulation 56:109, 1977

96. Corya BC, Rasmussen S, Knoebel S, Feigenbaum H, Black MJ: Echocardiocardiography in acute myocardial infarction. Am J Cardiol 36:1, 1975

97. Laurenceau J, Turcot J, Dumesnit J: Echocardiographic evaluation of ventricular wall thickness during acute coronary occlusions in dogs. Circulation (Suppl) 59, 60:II, 1979

98. Pandian N, Kerber R: Ultrasonic sonomicrometers vs 2-D echocardiography in the detection of transient myocardial dyskinesis. Circulation 62:III, 329, 1980

99. Weiss JL, Becker L, Bulkey B et al: Relationship of systolic thickening to transmural extent of myocardial infarction in the dog. Circulation (Suppl) 62:III, 328, 1980

100. Dodge HT, Sandler H, Ballen DW et al: The use of biplane angiocardiography for the measurement of left ventricular volume in man. Am Heart J 60:762, 1960

101. Dodge HT, Sandler H, Bailey WA et al: Usefulness and limitations of radiographic methods for determining left ventricular volume. Am J Cardiol 18:10, 1966

102. Sandler H, Dodge HT: The use of single plane angiocardiograms for the calculation of left ventricular volume in man. Am Heart J 75:325, 1968

103. Rakowski H, Martin RD, Popp RL: Left ventricular function: Assessment by wide angle two-dimensional ultrasonic sector scanning. Acta Med Scand (Suppl) 626:104, 1978

104. Carr K, Engler R, Forsythe J, Johnson A, Gosink B: Measurement of

left ventricular ejection fraction by mechanical cross-sectional echocardiography. Circulation 59:1196, 1979

105. Schiller N et al: Left ventricular volume from paired biplane two-dimensional echocardiography. Circulation 60:547, 1979
106. Wyatt H et al: Cross-sectional echocardiography. II. Analysis of mathematic models for quantifying volume of formalin fixed left ventricle. Circulation 61:1119, 1980
107. Blumgart HC, Weiss S: Studies on the velocity of blood flow: VII. The pulmonary circulation time in normal resting individuals. J Clin Invest 4:399, 1927
108. Prinzmetal M, Corday E, Spritzler RJ, Flieg W: Radiocardiography and its clinical applications. JAMA 139:617, 1949
109. Buja LM, Parkey RW, Dees JH et al: Morphologic correlates of technetium-99m stannous pyrophosphate imaging of acute myocardial infarcts in dogs. Circulation 52:596, 1975
110. Stokely EM, Buja LM, Lewis SE et al: Measurement of acute myocardial infarcts in dogs with 99m Tc-stannous pyrophosphate scintigrams. J Nucl Med 17:1, 1975
111. Zaret BL, Strauss HW, Martin ND et al: Noninvasive regional myocardial perfusion with radioactive potassium: Study of patients at rest, with exercise and during angina pectoris. N Engl J Med 288:809, 1973
112. Martin ND, Zaret BL, McGowan RL et al: Rubidium-81, a new myocardial scanning agent: Noninvasive regional myocardial perfusion scans at rest and exercise and comparison with potassium-43. Radiology 111:651, 1974
113. Wackers F, Sokole FB, Samson G et al: Value and limitations of thallium-201 scintigraphy in the acute phase of myocardial infarction. N Engl J Med 295:1, 1976
114. Bailey IK, Griffith LS, Rouleau J et al: Thallium-201 myocardial perfusion imaging at rest and during exercise: Comparative sensitivity to electrocardiography in coronary artery disease. Circulation 55:79, 1977
115. Ritchie JL, Trobaugh GB, Hamilton GW et al: Myocardial imaging with thallium-201 at rest and during exercise. Circulation 56:66, 1977
116. Botvinick EH, Taradash MR, Shames DM: Thallium-201 myocardial perfusion scintigraphy for the clinical clarification of normal, abnormal and equivocal electrocardiographic stress tests. Am J Cardiol 41:43, 1978
117. Schelbert HR, Verba JW, Johnson AD et al: Nontraumatic determination of left ventricular ejection fraction by radionuclide angiocardiography. Circulation 51:902, 1975
118. Marshall RC, Berger HJ, Costin JC et al: Assessment of cardiac performance with quantitative radionuclide angiocardiography: Sequential left ventricular ejection fraction, normalized left ventricular ejection rate and regional wall motion. Circulation 56:820, 1977
119. Jengo JA, Mena J, Blaufuss A et al: Evaluation of left ventricular function (ejection fraction and segmental wall motion) by single pass radioisotope angiography. Circulation 57:326, 1978
120. Berger HJ, Matthay RA, Loke J et al: Assessment of cardiac perfor-

mance with quantitative radionuclide angiocardiography: Right ventricular ejection fraction with reference to findings in chronic obstructive pulmonary disease. Am J Cardiol 41:897, 1978

121. Matthay R, Berger HJ, Loke J et al: Right and left ventricular performance in cystic fibrosis: Assessment by noninvasive radionuclide angiocardiography. Chest 72:407, 1977

122. Matthay R, Berger H, Gottschalk A et al: Effects of aminophylline on right and left ventricular performance in chronic obstructive pulmonary disease: Assessment by quantitative radionuclide angiocardiography. Am J Med 65:903, 1978

123. Reduto L, Berger H, Cohen LS et al: Sequential radionuclide assessment of left and right ventricular performance after acute transmural myocardial infarction. Ann Intern Med 89:441, 1978

124. Cohn JN, Guiha NH, Border MI et al: Right ventricular infarction. Clinical and hemodynamic features. Am J Cardiol 33:209, 1974

125. Polak JF, Kemper AJ, Bianco JA et al: A sensitive index of myocardial dysfunction in patients with coronary artery disease. J Nucl Med 23:471, 1982

126. Papapietro SE, Yester MV, Logic JR et al: Method for quantitative analysis of regional left ventricular function with first pass and gated blood pool scintigraphy. Am J Cardiol 47:618, 1981

127. Ratib O, Henze E, Schon H et al: Phase analysis of radionuclide ventriculograms for the detection of coronary artery disease. Am Heart J 104:1, 1982

128. Vos PH, Vossepoel AM, Pauwels EKJ: Quantitative assessment of wall motion in multiple-gated studies using temporal Fourier analysis. J Nucl Med 24:388, 1983

129. Lam W, Pavel D, Byron E et al: Radionuclide regurgitant index: Value and limitations. Am J Cardiol 47:292, 1981

130. Ashburn WL, Schelbert HR, Verba JW: Left ventricular ejection fraction: A review of several radinuclide angiographic approaches using the scintillation camera. Progr Cardiovasc Dis 20:267, 1978

131. Slutsky R, Karliner J, Ricci D et al: Response of left ventricular volume to exercise in man assessed by radionuclide equilibrium angiography. Circulation 60:565, 1979

132. Van Slyke DD, Neill JM: The determination of gases in blood and other solutions by vacuum extraction and manometric measurements. J Biol Chem 8:654, 1962

133. Gorlin R, Gorlin G: Hydraulic formula for calculation of area of stenotic mitral value, other valves and central circulatory shunts. Am Heart J 41:1, 1951

134. Cohen MV, Gorlin R: Modified orifice equation for the calculation of mitral valve area. Am Heart J 84:839, 1972

135. Grossman W: Cardiac Catheterization and Angiography, 2nd ed. Philadelphia, Lea & Febiger, 1980

136. Ganz W, Tamura K, Marcus HS et al: Measurement of coronary sinus blood flow by continuous thermodilution in man. Circulation 44:181, 1971

137. Rackley CE: Quantitative evaluation of left ventricular function by radiographic techniques. Circulation 54:862, 1976

138. Karliner JS, Peterson KL, Ross J Jr: Myocardial mechanics: Assessment of isovolumic and ejection phase indices of left ventricular performance. In Grossman W (ed): Cardiac Catheterization and Angiography, pp 188–206. Philadelphia, Lea & Febiger, 1974

139. Cohn PF, Gorlin R, Adams DF et al: Comparison of biplane and single-plane left ventriculography in patients with coronary artery disease. Am J Cardiol 33:1, 1974

140. Bove AA, Kreulen TH, Spann JF: Computer analysis of left ventricular dynamic geometry in man. Am J Cardiol 41:1239, 1978

141. Mangano DT: Preoperative assessment of cardiac catheterization data: Which are the most important parameters? Anesthesiology 53(3S):S105, 1980

142. White CW, Wright CB, Doty DB et al: Does visual interpretation of the coronary arteriogram predict the physiologic importance of a coronary stenosis? N Engl J Med 310:819, 1984

143. Alderman EL, Hamilton KK, Silverman J et al: Anatomically flexible, computer-assisted reporting system for coronary angiography. Am J Cardiol 49:1208, 1982

144. Chazov EI, Matveeva LS, Mazaev AV et al: Intracoronary administration of fibrinolysin in acute MI. Ter Arkh 4:8, 1976

145. Chazov EI, Lakin KM: Anticoagulants and fibrinolytics. Chicago, Yearbook Medical Publishers, 1980

146. Rentrop P: Mortality and functional changes after intracoronary streptokinase infusion. Circulation 66:II-335, 1982

147. Schwarz F, Schuler G, Katus H: Intracoronary thrombolysis in myocardial infarction: Duration of ischemia as a major determinant of late results after recanalization. Am J Cardiol 50:933, 1982

148. Gruentzig AR, Senning A, Siegenthaler WE et al: Nonoperative dilatation of coronary artery stenosis: percutaneous transluminal coronary angioplasty. N Engl J Med 301:62, 1979

149. Goldberg S, Urban P, Greenspan A: Combination therapy for evolving myocardial infarction: Intracoronary thrombolysis and percutaneous transluminal angioplasty. Am J Med 72:994, 1982

150. Meyer J, Merz W, Schmitz H: Percutaneous transluminal coronary angioplasty immediately after intracoronary streptolysis of transmural myocardial infarction. Circulation 66:905, 1982

151. Hartzler GO, Rutherford BD, McConhay DR: Percutaneous transluminal coronary angioplasty with and without thrombolytic therapy for treatment of acute myocardial infarction. Am Heart J 1067:965, 1983

152. Cowley MJ, Vetrovec GW, Lewis SA et al: Coronary angioplasty of multiple vessels: Acute and long term results. Circulation 70 (abstract) (suppl II):322, 1984

153. Dorros G, Cowley MJ, Simpson J et al: Percutaneous transluminal coronary angioplasty: Report of complications from the National Heart, Lung, and Blood Institute PTCA Registry. Circulation 67:723, 1983

154. Higgins CB, Lanzer P, Stark D et al: Imaging by nuclear magnetic resonance in patients with chronic ischemic heart disease. Circulation 69:523, 1984

155. Ordidge RJ, Mansfield P, Doyle M et al: "Real-time" moving images by NMR. In Witcofski RL, Karstaedt N, Partain CL (eds): Proceedings of the International Symposium in NMR Imaging, pp 80–92. Winston-Salem, NC, Bowman Gray School of Medicine Press, 1982
156. DeLayre JL, Ingwall JS, Malloy C et al: Gated sodium-23 nuclear magnetic resonance images of an isolated perfused working rat heart. Science 212:935, 1981

John M. Jackson
Patti S. Klein
Stephen J. Thomas

2 | Preoperative Assessment of the Patient with Valvular Heart Disease

Few outcome data exist for perioperative risk in patients with valvular heart disease (VHD), probably because definitive disease-specific or perioperative criteria are difficult to obtain in this population. Acute hypertension resulting in a precipitously accentuated "V" wave (mitral valve regurgitation [MR]), tachycardia-induced hypotension in the patient with aortic stenosis (AS), and oliguria in the hypovolemic patient with aortic regurgitation (AR) are potential perioperative episodes familiar to clinicians experienced in the management of patients with VHD who undergo noncardiac surgery. These are transient perturbations, too ephemeral (*i.e.*, usually immediately treatable) to define severity and, thus, potential risk status. Without that objective data, it becomes necessary to extrapolate known risk factors for perioperative cardiac morbidity in VHD patients to the noncardiac surgical population. Potential risk factors must be gleaned from the clinical history, physical examination, and pathophysiologic derangements characteristic of individual valvular lesions.

VHD AND PERIOPERATIVE RISK: PRE- AND POST-GOLDMAN

Initially, only aortic valvular disease (AS and AR) was associated with increased perioperative mortality,[1] not related conditions, such as dysrhythmias and concurrent ischemic heart disease. Goldman and colleagues demonstrated the significance of these independent risk factors in their landmark study.[2]

For patients with all forms of VHD, the perioperative risk of developing new, or worse, congestive heart failure (CHF) was reported to be approximately 20%. The only independent predictors of postoperative congestive failure in these patients, however, were the same as those in patients with nonvalvular disease—preoperative symptoms confirmed by physical examination. Aortic stenosis was the only valvular disease found to be an independent risk factor for perioperative cardiac morbidity in VHD patients with and without CHF. When AS was associated with postoperative congestive failure, it was thought to reflect "the unique difficulties in perioperative fluid management" specific to this group of patients. Aortic stenosis also resulted in 14-fold higher perioperative mortality. Similarly, mitral regurgitation (MR) (grade II/VI or greater) predisposed higher mortality, although MR was not considered an independent risk factor. The increase in mortality was attributed to the frequent association of MR with other independent clinical risk factors, specifically an S3 gallop (S3G), jugular venous distention (JVD), or a recent myocardial infarction (MI).

The first of Goldman's findings was reassuring news for the clinical anesthesiologist. Specifically, there are good prospective data suggesting that the severity of a patient's preoperative symptoms correlate with the relative degree of perioperative cardiac risk. Therefore, it is initially unnecessary to incur either the morbidity (negligible) or the expense (not at all negligible) associated with the use of invasive and noninvasive diagnostic techniques in assessing patients with VHD. Perhaps even more reassuring is that Goldman's observation parallels well-established data demonstrating that the significance of symptoms in patients with VHD helps to quantify the underlying inotropic state of the myocardium.

Other than age and the influence of recent MI, the independent clinical risk factors identified by Goldman are those indicative of cardiac failure (S3 gallop, JVD). Signs and symptoms of CHF probably are accurate indicators of a presumably depressed and anesthetically vulnerable myocardium in patients with ischemic heart disease, but similarly severe symptoms may not correlate with the underlying contractile state of the myocardium in patients with VHD, particularly those with AS and mitral stenosis (MS). Such symptoms often indicate characteristic, deleterious imbalances between inotropic state and prevailing ventricular loading conditions. Appropriate hemodynamic provocation (*e.g.*, tachycardia accompanying appendicitis in a previously well-compensated patient with MS) would alter the ventricle's prevailing load and precipitate pulmonary edema, necessitating emergency surgery. Neither the tachycardia nor the inflamed appendix would directly or indirectly depress the inotropic state of the left ventricle (LV), which would remain normal. CHF might accompany contractile dysfunction in patients with end-stage pulmonary hypertension and biventricular failure secondary to uncorrected MS or MR.

THE MYOCARDIUM IN VHD: SYSTOLIC PERFORMANCE VS. INOTROPY

The primary abnormalities among patients with VHD occur in loading conditions. Ross has developed a popular load-dependent model that distinguishes the performance of the heart as a pump (its systolic function or ejection performance) from the intrinsic inotropic state of the myocardium (inotropy or contractility).[3] Central to its use is the role of ventricular afterload in the regulation of myocardial performance, specifically, the inverse relationship between the prevailing afterload and stroke volume of the ventricle (Fig. 2-1).

This relationship is represented in Figure 2-2 as an experimentally constructed LV pressure-volume loop where afterload is progressively increased while preload is held constant. Normally, LV stroke volume is maintained (normalized ejection performance) by compensatory increases in preload due to the Frank–Starling mechanism. Increased afterload in the presence of limited or exhausted pre-

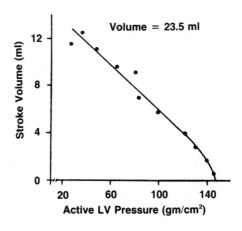

FIGURE 2-1. Plot of stroke volume versus maximum generated left ventricular systolic pressure, demonstrating the inverse force–velocity relationship. During construction of this curve, end-diastolic volume was held constant. *(Burns JW, Covell JW, Ross J Jr: Mechanics of isotonic left ventricular contractions. AM J Physiol 224:725, 1973)*

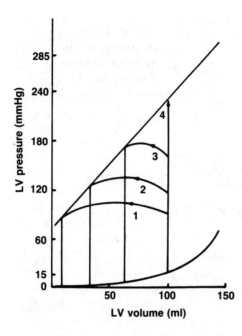

FIGURE 2-2. Pressure-volume loops demonstrating the fall in stroke volume that occurs with increases in afterload when preload is artificially held constant. *(Ross J Jr: Afterload mismatch in aortic and mitral valve disease: Implications for surgical therapy. J Am Coll Cardiol 5:811, 1985)*

load can decrease ejection performance, causing failure of the heart at a time when myocardial contractility may be normal.[3] Conversely, favorable loading conditions (abnormally low ventricular afterload) could preserve the heart's ejection performance and thereby mask an intrinsically depressed myocardium.

AORTIC REGURGITATION AND MITRAL REGURGITATION: VOLUME OVERLOAD OF THE LEFT VENTRICLE

Pathophysiology

Aortic regurgitation (AR) and mitral regurgitation (MR) both produce chronic volume overloading of the LV.[4] In chronic AR, preload increases in direct proportion to the amount of regurgitant volume determined by the regurgitant orifice size, the diastolic time interval, and the pressure gradient between the aorta and the LV throughout diastole. This progressive use of preload reserve allows the LV to normalize stroke volume (systolic performance) despite concurrent deterioration in intrinsic contractile function (inotropy). Wall stress (pressure × volume/wall thickness) eventually increases because cavitary enlargement (V) predominates over wall thickening in the pathophysiology of volume-induced, serial replication of sarcomeres (eccentric hypertrophy). Normally, higher wall stress would decrease stroke volume, but the eccentrically dilated ventricle maintains forward flow due to its higher preload (the rightward shift on the volume axis) (Fig. 2-3).

Concurrent inotropic deterioration becomes apparent when the ventricle reaches the limit of its eccentric enlargement. Deprived of further compensation by the Starling mechanism, the ventricle fails to deliver a normal stroke volume when faced with the higher afterload. Heightened sympathetic outflow and accompanying tachycardia help to maintain cardiac output during declining stroke volume. Tachycardia also minimizes the regurgitant flow per beat by shortening diastole. Simultaneously, the time for perfusion of the enlarged myocardial mass is reduced. Despite this pathology, angina pectoris occurs in few patients having chronic AR, perhaps because the increased work performed by the enlarged heart is expended in the relatively

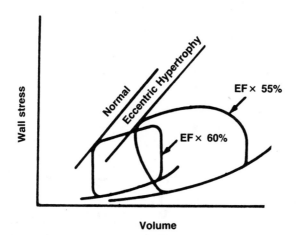

Volume

FIGURE 2-3. Adaptation to chronic volume overload in aortic regurgitation. A shift down and to the right of the diastolic pressure-volume relationship (compliance) allows maintenance of stroke volume in the face of slightly elevated wall stress. *(Ross J Jr: Afterload mismatch in aortic and mitral valve disease: Implications for surgical therapy. J Am Coll Cardiol 5:811, 1985)*

energy-efficient process of fiber shortening, rather than to the more oxygen-costly effort of pressure generation.

Patients with acute AR are threatened by very different pathophysiologic constraints. Large regurgitant volumes are delivered to a nondilated ventricle having normal inotropic and compliance properties. With no rightward shift in the ventricular diastolic pressure-volume curve, severe regurgitation and the resultant large end-diastolic volumes precipitously increase ventricular end-diastolic pressure (Fig. 2-4). As in patients with chronic AR, severe retrograde flow decreases net forward flow, resulting in a subnormal diastolic pressure and compensatory tachycardia that potentially compromises coronary perfusion. The potential for ischemia is greater in patients with acute AR, however, because concurrent and precipitous increases in the LV end-diastolic pressure threaten to further impede coronary perfusion (assuming that coronary perfusion pressure is related to

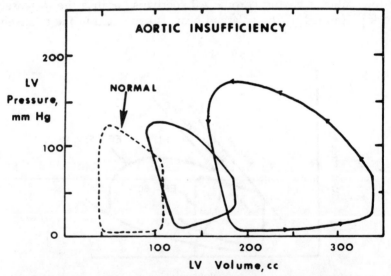

FIGURE 2-4.   Pressure-volume loops of acute and chronic aortic regurgitation (AR) compared with normal pressure volume. Acute AR (middle loop) illustrates a continuation of the normal diastolic-volume relationship, with very high LV end-diastolic pressure. Compare that to the downward shift noted in chronic AVR where LV end-diastolic pressure is only minimally elevated, despite doubling or tripling ventricular volume. *(Redrawn from Jackson JM, Thomas SJ, Lowenstein E: Anesthetic management of patients with valvular heart disease. Semin Anesth 1:239, 1982)*

the difference between diastolic pressures in the aorta and LV) and simultaneously elevate myocardial oxygen demand (increased end-diastolic wall tension).

Mitral Regurgitation

In chronic MR, the LV wall stress–volume relationship shifts to the right; that is, the ventricle dilates (Fig. 2-5A). The only significant difference between this and AR is that LV wall stress is not increased, but probably is decreased, due to the regurgitant leak in the left atrium. The decrease in wall stress combined with the use of preload reserve may actually permit the LV to deliver a supranormal stroke volume having a higher than normal ejection fraction, suggesting enhanced systolic performance. The ventricle's intrinsic inotropic state is imperiled, however, by the eccentric enlargement accompanying MR. In Figure 2-5B, such occult myocardial depression is signified by the normal ejection fraction (50%) and the normal (*i.e.*, not increased) stroke volume.

Because of the early, vigorous retrograde ejection into the low-pressure left atrium, ventricular systole lacks an isovolumetric phase. Favorable loading conditions thereby enhance the ejection performance of an intrinsically depressed myocardium. In patients undergoing valve replacement, this occult myocardial depression often manifests postoperatively when the ventricular systolic performance declines (see Fig. 2-5B) in response to the newly elevated afterload imposed by the competent mitral prosthesis (afterload mismatch).[4]

The clinical symptoms of MR develop more gradually than those of the other valvular lesions. Patients with mild disease may be asymptomatic. Apparent symptoms are those of LV dysfunction, which are determined by LV status and the size of the regurgitant volume. Patients may complain of fatigue, weight loss, and weakness consistent with low cardiac output, or have symptoms of pulmonary congestion. There may be associated symptoms of right ventricular failure. Untreated, these symptoms correlate with a 5-year mortality rate of 50%. Complications include endocarditis, embolic events, and atrial tachyarrhythmias.

Implications for Risk Assessment

The prognostic significance of preoperative symptoms of CHF may have a clear pathophysiologic basis, particularly in patients with

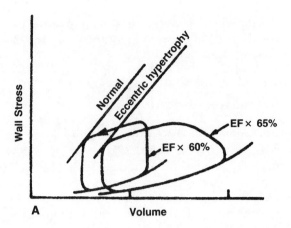

A Volume

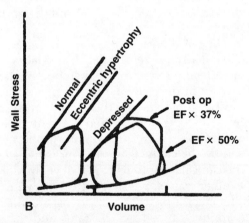

B Volume

FIGURE 2-5. Pressure-volume loops for chronic mitral regurgitation (MVR).
(A) Displacement of the diastolic pressure-volume relationship down and to the
right, accommodating the increase in left ventricular volume. There is no increase
in wall stress and no period of isovolumic systole, since blood is ejected directly
to the left atrium with the onset of contraction. (B) Because of these ideal
loading conditions, ejection fraction can be maintained, even in the face of
depressed myocardial contractility. When afterload is increased, in this case by
value replacement, ejection fraction falls as a result of the afterload mismatch.
*(Ross J Jr: Afterload mismatch in aortic and mitral valve disease: Implications for
surgical therapy. J Am Coll Cardiol 5:811, 1985)*

chronic regurgitant disease. Preoperative symptoms in these patients indicate the likelihood of an intrinsically depressed myocardium whose systolic performance may be exquisitely sensitive to loading conditions. Prophylaxis or treatment of predictable afterload stresses associated with surgical or anesthetic interventions (aortic cross clamping, failure to blunt reflex vasoconstriction, inappropriate treatment with exogenous vasoconstrictors) is necessary. Additionally, intravascular volume must be maintained (rightward shift of pressure-volume curve) to maximize forward flow and to ensure adequate end-organ perfusion. Parenteral vasodilators or a vasodilating anesthetic agent or technique often are critical adjuncts in balancing an appropriately full intravasculature against the vulnerability of an intrinsically depressed myocardium. This is particularly true in the immediate postoperative period, when various adverse trends (hypothermia, pain, return of sympathetic reflexes) may combine to create an acute afterload mismatch.

A clinically important corollary of this shift in the pressure–volume relationship is LV high diastolic compliance in patients with chronic AR (large end-diastolic volumes associated with normal or only minimal elevations in the LV end-diastolic pressure). Although this property may minimize discrepancies between the central venous and pulmonary capillary wedge pressures, cardiac output must be monitored by pulmonary-artery (PA) catheter to capture iatrogenically induced (positional, mechanical, pharmacological) afterload stresses.

Patients with acute AR do not often require noncardiac surgery, but may undergo a noncardiac procedure prior to emergent valve replacement (*e.g.*, for trauma, embolic complications). Hemodynamic decompensation often is severe in these cases and usually reflects the magnitude of LV distention during diastole and the accompanying ischemic threat to previously normal myocardium. Extremely precarious hemodynamic stability may be achieved within very narrow constraints of heart rate, blood pressure, and intravascular filling pressures. The priority is to minimize the regurgitant volume, because it is the final, common pathway leading to simultaneous hypotension, tachycardia, and myocardial oxygen demand–supply imbalance. The strategy is to avoid bradycardia and its attendant prolongation of the diastolic interval for retrograde flow. Various nondepressant induction techniques might promote bradycardia simply by withdrawal of sympathetic outflow.

Specific, otherwise hemodynamically desirable agents (*e.g.*, narcotics) also could potentiate bradycardia through a vagotonic mechanism. Consequently, a reliable method of sequential pacing should be established before induction of general anesthesia. A PA catheter with pacing capability can be used. One limitation of the PA catheter technique is that the pulmonary capillary wedge pressures may seriously underestimate the LV end-diastolic pressure when the regurgitant volume is large, because the precipitously rising LV end-diastolic pressure prematurely closes the mitral valve.[5] Thus the LV may continue to receive substantial diastolic inflow from the aorta at a time when the mitral valve is closed and the pulmonary capillary wedge pressure cannot approximate the end-diastolic pressure.

Echocardiography can quantify the ventricular distention, and provide useful information about systolic function, wall-motion abnormalities, and severity of valvular insufficiency. Pulmonary artery pressure monitoring also is probably warranted in most patients with chronic MR undergoing major noncardiac surgical procedures, particularly those with end-stage disease whose advanced age, severe myocardial dysfunction, or otherwise debilitated condition may preclude their candidacy for valve replacement. Pulmonary artery pressures at, or close to, systemic levels may indicate severe risk of acute right heart failure which would be exacerbated by even the slightest degree of volume overload. In less severely compromised patients, the wedge tracing should be checked periodically for evidence of acute changes in the configuration of the regurgitant V wave. Although its absolute height is unreliable for quantifying regurgitant flow, relative changes in V wave severity may be helpful in monitoring the responses to beneficial and deleterious changes in afterload.

Given the wedge tracing's limitations as a real-time quantifier of retrograde flow, noninvasive measurements of disease severity assume greater importance in the preoperative evaluation of patients with MR. Doppler echocardiography, by detecting systolic turbulence in the left atrium (representing the regurgitant jet), provides a semiquantitative approximation of the degree of valvular insufficiency.[6–8] The sensitivity of this technique increases with both severity of the disease and the etiology of regurgitation.[6] For example, mitral regurgitation of rheumatic origin is easier to diagnose than that due to mitral valve prolapse or a cleft leaflet. False positives are common, however, because Doppler echocardiographic analysis can distinguish among absent, mild, or severe regurgitation, but it cannot accurately quantify the regurgitant fraction.[9]

Of the commonly available noninvasive techniques, radionuclide angiography most accurately quantifies the regurgitant volume, and is considered the standard for preoperative assessment of patients having severe symptoms and of candidates for valve replacement. Results correlate well with regurgitant volumes determined at the time of diagnostic catheterization. The cineangiographic severity of MR commonly is graded in values of 1 + to 4 + as described below:[10]

1 + = not enough contrast to outline left atrium
2 + = faint outline of left atrium with contrast without equilibration between LV and left atrium
3 + = rapid outline of left atrium with equilibration between LV and left atrium after the third systole
4 + = rapid outline of left atrium with equilibration between LV and left atrium before the third systole

Intraoperative management of asymptomatic patients with regurgitant VHD should maintain the compensatory mechanisms (adequate preload, decreased afterload) that preserve systolic function in the face of progressive LV enlargement. The natural history of chronic aortic regurgitation (75% 5-year and 50% 10-year, survival, without therapy) is such that minimally symptomatic or asymptomatic patients already may have significant cardiomegaly and varying degrees of intrinsic contractile dysfunction. Preoperative evaluation by the consulting cardiologist may include a determination of the LV ejection fraction interpreted relative to its known afterload sensitivity. More important than a single determination of such an ejection phase index is any demonstrable trend in serial determinations. The latter information is worth pursuing with echocardiography or radionuclide angiography to pinpoint the earliest stages of contractile dysfunction.[11–14]

AORTIC STENOSIS: PRESSURE OVERLOAD OF THE LEFT VENTRICLE

As in patients with chronic regurgitant disease, the natural history of AS is one of a decades-long latency period preceding the appearance of one or more of the classic symptoms of angina, syncope, or CHF. Symptomatic patients share a uniformly poor prognosis with medical therapy (Fig. 2-6) and should undergo valve replacement as soon as possible.

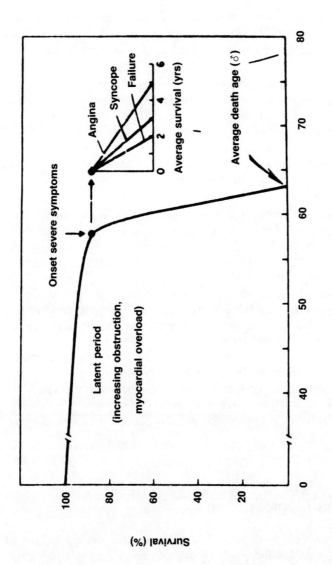

FIGURE 2-6. Nonoperative natural history of aortic stenosis. *(Ross J Jr, and Braunwald, E: Aortic stenosis. Circulation 38[Suppl.V]:61, 1968, by permission of the American Heart Association)*

Pathophysiology

The LV has a chronic pressure overload in AS, which produces disparities between the ventricle's systolic performance and underlying inotropic state that are qualitatively similar to those encountered in patients with regurgitant disease. In animals, chronic pressure overload in the form of supravalvular constriction is a specific stimulus to the parallel replication of sarcomeres,[15,16] and results in concentric ventricular hypertrophy (as in regurgitant disease with hypertrophy) (Fig. 2-7).

Although the classic symptoms of AS (angina, syncope) suggest systolic dysfunction, there is increasing evidence that the ventricle's underlying inotropic state often is normal or supranormal, and that hypertrophically-induced diastolic dysfunction predominates in most patients. These conditions are apparent in the pressure-volume loop analysis of the pressure overloaded ventricle (Fig. 2-8A).

Compared with the prehypertrophy control loop A, the ventricle affected by chronic pressure overload, loop B, achieves much higher peak end-systolic pressures at a comparable end-diastolic volume. Maintaining stroke volume, the diseased ventricle generates this higher peak systolic pressure during isovolumic systole despite valvular outflow obstruction (*i.e.*, normal/supranormal systolic function). A wall-stress versus volume analysis shows that myocardial contractility usually is normal, not supranormal (Fig.2-8B).

The concurrent development of diastolic dysfunction is evident in the increased slope of the diastolic limb of the pressure-volume loop. This increased slope demonstrates decreased diastolic compliance, a property generally associated with concentric hypertrophy and also observed with LV hypertrophy due to hypertension and hypertrophic cardiomyopathy.[17-20] From echocardiographic studies, it appears that the deterioration in diastolic compliance parallels the absolute degree of ventricular hypertrophy (Fig. 2-9).[21]

The reasons for the apparently constant relationship between concentric ventricular hypertrophy and deteriorated diastolic compliance are unknown. However, ischemia-induced abnormalities of myocardial relaxation may contribute to hypertrophy-induced diastolic dysfunction.[22] The determinants of myocardial oxygen demand (*e.g.*, wall tension and contractility) are not exclusively systolic phenomena. Diastolic relaxation also is an energy-requiring process, during which myoplasmic calcium located in the interdigitating myofilaments during systole is returned during diastole (largely by ATP-consuming pumps) to membrane storage depots located in the inner aspect of the sarcolemma, the mitochondria, and the sarco-

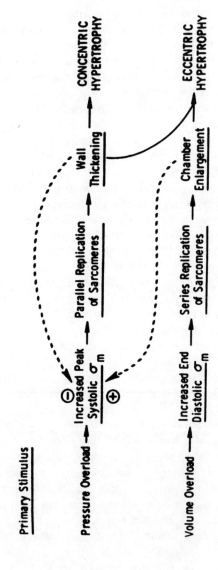

FIGURE 2-7. Ventricular responses to chronic pressure and volume overload. (See text.) (Grossman W, Jones D, McLaurin LP: *Wall stress and patterns of hypertrophy in the human left ventricle. J Clin Invest 56:56, 1975*)

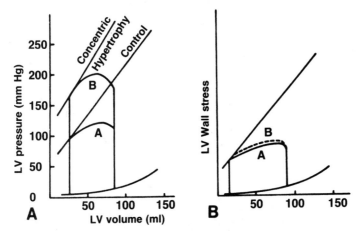

FIGURE 2-8.   Pressure-volume loops and end-systolic pressure-volume relationship (ESPVR) with chronic pressure overload. (*A*) With increased intraventricular pressure, stroke volume is maintained and the ESPVR is shifted up and to the left, suggesting increased contractility. (*B*) Substitution of wall stress for LV pressure, indicating normal, unchanged contractility. *(Ross J Jr: Afterload mismatch in aortic and mitral valve disease: Implications for surgical therapy. J Am Coll Cardiol 5:811, 1985)*

plasmic reticulum. Patients with AS are uniquely at risk for a potentially imbalanced myocardial oxygen demand–supply relationship. Basal myocardial oxygen requirements are elevated by an increase in overall muscle mass, and systolic oxygen requirements increase in proportion to the degree of wall tension required to overcome the valvular obstruction, affecting demand. Hypertrophy is not completely deleterious to myocardial energetics, however, because of the inverse relationship between systolic wall tension and myocardial wall thickness: wall tension = P × V/h. Pressure overload (V) directly increases myocardial wall tension, a major determinant of myocardial oxygen demand, but also stimulates concentric hypertrophy (h), which tends to minimize the level of wall tension developed for any degree of valvular obstruction (P). Accordingly, one hypothesis[23] for the onset of systolic dysfunction in patients with AS is that hypertrophy fails to keep pace with the degree of obstruction, resulting in increased wall tension and decreased stroke volume (afterload mismatch).[4]

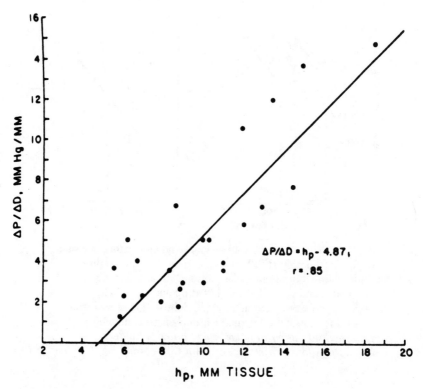

FIGURE 2-9. The relationship between wall thickness (h_p) and chamber stiffness (P/D), the inverse of compliance. *(Grossman W, McLaurin P, Moos SP, et al: Wall thickness and diastolic properties of the left ventricle. Circulation 49:129, 1974)*

Coronary perfusion also may be compromised by both anatomic and hemodynamic factors. Patients with an LV pressure overload have an increased incidence of atherosclerotic coronary artery disease.[24,25] Furthermore, myocardial hypertrophy often is associated with a failure of concurrent, proportional growth in the cross-sectional area of the coronary vasculature.[26,27] Hemodynamic impediments to coronary blood flow also impose risk. Perfusion of the deep subendocardial layers of the hypertrophied myocardium is critically dependent on adequate time for diastolic coronary perfusion. Greater degrees of valvular obstruction prolong systolic ejection time and correspondingly reduce diastolic time for coronary perfusion. An important corollary of the ventricle's poor diastolic compliance is an inevitable narrowing of the approximate coronary perfusion pressure.

Implications for Risk Assessment

A detailed clinical history and physical examination are the initial steps in assessing noncardiac perioperative risk. Elderly patients with a systolic ejection murmur may appear to have AS and require noninvasive hemodynamic testing to differentiate the diagnosis.

Generally, the risk assessment priorities in patients with AS are determinations of the presence or absence of symptoms, transaortic gradient, and LV function. Although normal contractility is the rule, establishing LV function is important because there is a subset of patients who may exhibit depressed contractility, most likely due to subendocardial ischemia. For symptomatic patients being evaluated before valve replacement surgery, the ejection fraction has predictive value only if it is normal preoperatively. Patients with a preoperatively depressed ejection fraction may recover ventricular function after valve replacement, their low ejection fraction likely being due to inadequate hypertrophy[23] and consequent elevated wall tension or afterload mismatch. Valve replacement removes the afterload stress, allowing the stroke volume and ejection fraction to increase.

For patients presenting for noncardiac surgery, noninvasive testing usually includes M-mode, two-dimensional, and Doppler echocardiography. Although M-mode echocardiography cannot determine the severity of obstruction, it can distinguish several of the characteristic pathologic findings of the disease, including LV hypertrophy, increased LV end-diastolic pressure, and aortic dilatation.[28] M-mode studies also can be used to assess LV function. Two-dimensional echocardiography may provide additional information about the degree of stenosis, but has limited accuracy in patients with only moderate obstruction.[29-31]

Doppler studies accurately detect the presence of AS by identification of turbulent blood flow distal to the stenotic lesion. The peak gradient across the valve may be derived and correlates well with that determined by invasive catheterization (Fig. 2-10).[32] The severity of stenosis is determined by Doppler analysis, using the LV ejection time and the change in configuration of the systolic Doppler signal as the stenosis worsens.[6] The presence of a significant gradient (> 50 mmHg) in an asymptomatic patient does not indicate catheterization or valve replacement, although invasive monitoring is often helpful for procedures likely to be associated with significant volume shifts.

The goals of intravascular fluid therapy in patients with AS must be clearly defined, because these patients are at significantly increased risk for postoperative CHD.[2] Since this is a disease whose unifying pathophysiologic derangement is that of diastolic dysfunc-

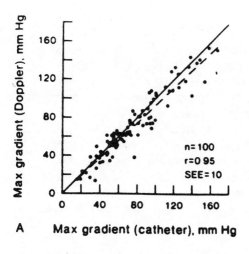

A

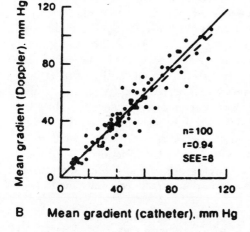

B

FIGURE 2-10. Correlation of aortic valve gradient determined by cardiac catheterization and Doppler echocardiography (A = maximum, B = mean) in 100 patients with aortic stenosis. The solid lines are lines of identity, the dotted lines are regression lines. *(Currie PJ et al: Instantaneous pressure gradient: A simultaneous Doppler and dual catheter correlative study. J Am Coll Cardiol 7:803, 1986)*

tion, specifically a noncompliant or "stiff" LV, patients require a higher than normal LV end-diastolic pressure to maintain forward flow, adequate blood pressure, and end-organ perfusion. The elevated LV end-diastolic pressure also opposes the normally large contribution of passive diastolic filling to LV end-diastolic volume,[17] making these patients critically dependent on atrial systole for maintaining adequate ventricular preload. The higher LV end-diastolic pressure (end-diastolic volume) allows the LV to achieve the wall-tension development required to eject a normal stroke volume in the presence of the stenotic aortic valve. The higher LV end-diastolic pressure probably also impedes an already compromised blood supply to the subendocardium, placing the hypertrophied ventricle at risk for ischemic dysfunction (both systolic and diastolic). This last possibility should be considered when the LV end-diastolic pressure further increases in the absence of other evidence of intravascular overload, or increases in response to potentially ischemia-producing stimuli (transient hypotension, tachycardia).[33] This exacerbation of an already increased LV end-diastolic pressure may be the only objective index of myocardial ischemia in patients having pre-existing, hypertrophy-induced ST segment abnormalities.

Symptomatic patients with AS are not candidates for elective noncardiac surgery and should undergo an initial, noninvasive evaluation, followed by cardiac catheterization. Although some clinicians disavow the need for invasive hemodynamic evaluation,[34,35] others favor catheterization in order to:

1. Assess the mechanical severity of the disease
2. Identify concurrent coronary artery disease
3. Determine the presence of aortic insufficiency
4. Assess LV function

Catheterization findings may be normal when the aortic valve area is > 1 cm^2; smaller areas usually are associated with a systolic pressure gradient across the valve. The Gorlin formula dictates that the gradient across a stenotic valve varies with the square of the cardiac output.[36] A small gradient may underestimate the severity of disease if the flow at the time of measurement is low. A gradient > 50 mmHg in the presence of a normal cardiac output indicates severe disease.[37] However, the calculated valve area is a better indicator of stenotic severity than is the gradient across the valve.

Symptomatic patients are candidates for valve replacement when they have hemodynamic evidence of severe disease (valve orifice area < 0.75 cm^2); asymptomatic patients are candidates when there is evidence of progressive LV dysfunction. Because LV function improves perioperatively (despite depressed preoperative ejection fractions), surgical prophylaxis for developing dysfunction is not recommended in asymptomatic patients.[38]

Elderly patients with symptomatic AS have a particularly poor prognosis (*i.e.*, survival rates of 57% and 37%, respectively, for the first and second year after the onset of symptoms[39]). Age alone does not contraindicate aortic valve replacement,[40] although recent studies report an increased incidence of neurologic events and increased mortality rates after aortic valve replacement for AS in patients older than 70 years.[41-43] Emergency surgery, endocarditis, reoperation, and coronary artery disease (CAD) also are risk factors in aortic valve replacement, for both AS and aortic insufficiency.[44]

Balloon valvuloplasty is a new and largely investigational technique, potentially useful in treating patients with critical AS who refuse valve replacement and those excluded from surgery.[11] The procedure relieves valvular obstruction in most subjects, but has been tested primarily in elderly patients with calcific AS.[45] It may have a role in relieving aortic obstruction before noncardiac surgery.[46]

MITRAL VALVE STENOSIS: VOLUME UNDERLOAD OF THE LEFT VENTRICLE

Mitral valve stenosis (MS) is primarily rheumatic in origin. Twenty-five percent of presenting patients have pure MS and 40% have combined MS and MR.[11] A latent period of 10 to 20 years follows an episode of acute rheumatic fever, during which time patients are asymptomatic. Once symptoms develop, they are rapidly progressive, resulting in pulmonary congestion and, if untreated, pulmonary hypertension and secondary right ventricular failure.[47,48] Symptom onset to severe disability averages approximately 7 years.[49]

Pathophysiology

The normal adult mitral valve has an area of 4 to 6 cm². A loss of 2 cm² requires an increase in the transvalvular pressure gradient to maintain normal blood flow. Mild disease exists with an area of 1.5 to 2.5 cm²; moderate disease with one of 1.1 to 1.5 cm².[47] Critical mitral stenosis exists when the area decreases to 0.6 to 1.0 cm², at which time the pressure gradient across the valve (left atrial pressure–LV end-diastolic pressure) becomes as high as 20 mmHg to maintain a normal cardiac output.

The transvalvular pressure gradient is closely linked to heart rate.[36] For a constant valve area, the pressure gradient is directly proportional to the square of the ratio of cardiac output divided by the diastolic filling time. Consequently, tachycardia, which compromises diastolic filling time and results in large increases in transvalvular pressure gradient, can easily precipitate pulmonary edema.

During MS, the LV's altered load, along with secondary or compensatory responses to this altered load, may induce an abrupt and dramatic difference between the patient's symptoms and underlying inotropic state. For example, myocardial contractility usually is normal in patients with MS,[50-54] but the conditions necessitating noncardiac surgery may precipitate an episode of acute pulmonary edema by increasing heart rate. This clinical presentation reflects only the hydraulic principles governing flow across the valve and does not indicate acute deterioration in the underlying inotropic state. In some patients, the underloaded ventricle's fixed stroke volume activates a reflex sympathetic response and increases systemic vascular resistance,[50] thereby depressing ejection phase indices. The distinction again is one of altered load. Systolic function is depressed because the inotropically normal myocardium is simultaneously underloaded (stenotic mitral valve) and afterload-stressed (high systemic vascular resistance), that is, an afterload mismatch.

Right ventricular contractile function also is normal in most patients with MS, even those with moderate pulmonary hypertension.[55] However, the right ventricle is a primarily high-volume, low-pressure pump, and an afterload mismatch due to long-standing or severe pulmonary hypertension (PAS > 70 mmHg) will cause contractile failure. Ultimately, the right ventricle will distend, producing secondary tricuspid or, rarely, pulmonary regurgitation.

Limited ventricular filling at the level of the stenotic mitral valve also contributes to chronically elevated left atrial pressure, attributable to restricted forward flow. These high left atrial pressures are transmitted back to the lungs, causing vascular engorgement and eventually increasing pulmonary venous, capillary, and pulmonary arterial pressures. Chronic pulmonary hypertension can result in reactive pulmonary vasoconstriction and permanent, obliterative changes in the pulmonary vascular bed. As long as patients remain in sinus rhythm, the brief atrial contraction helps to minimize the mean left atrial pressure at values lower than possible without the sinus mechanism. As disease progresses, diastolic filling time becomes more important than atrial systole in preserving forward flow. Tachycardia, not the loss of atrial contraction, is primarily responsible for the hemodynamic decompensation associated with rapid atrial fibrillation.

Passive or retrograde changes in the pulmonary vasculature may ultimately cause significant changes in pulmonary function in patients with mitral stenosis. The lungs manifest "brown induration" that results from parenchymal hemorrhage and secondary hemosiderosis. Mitral valve stenosis is associated with a marked decrease in lung compliance that increases the work of breathing and redistributes blood flow away from the base to the apices, resulting in ventilation-perfusion (V/Q) mismatch.[56,57] All aspects of lung function are affected. Lung volumes and flow rates progressively decline as disease worsens. The ventilatory defects parallel increases in pulmonary artery pressure and pulmonary vascular resistance. The vascular changes in MS correlate with changes in pulmonary artery pressure. Changes in pulmonary capillary wedge pressure vary inversely with changes in lung compliance measured during tidal volume breathing (*i.e.*, dynamic compliance).[57,58] Static lung measurements reveal abnormal elastic properties of the lungs, with a loss of recoil at smaller volumes because of vascular engorgement, and increased recoil at high volumes due to fibrosis.[58] Respiratory muscle dysfunction may occur,[59] and a reduced vital capacity may indicate impending congestive heart failure.[60] Resting arterial blood gases reveal normocarbia (or slight hypocarbia) and hypoxia that progresses with increasing disease severity. Diffusing capacity is impaired, and the severity of changes in pulmonary vascular resistance parallels a failure to increase diffusing capacity with increased oxygen uptake.

Implications for Risk Assessment

No current data suggest that patients with MS are at any increased risk for perioperative cardiac complications after noncardiac surgery. Unlike other valvular diseases, preoperative pump dysfunction (except in isolated or end-stage disease) is uncommon in patients with MS, perhaps because symptoms appear earlier in these patients. Unlike mitral regurgitation, the natural history of patients having mitral stenosis requires surgical treatment at an earlier stage, so these patients often meet accepted criteria for elective valve replacement long before the occurrence of irreversible, dysfunctional changes in myocardium. Preoperatively, congestive symptoms may be attributable to associated pulmonary dysfunction. Although pulmonary function tests will quantify the severity of lung disease and help to predict postoperative morbidity and mortality, they may be little help in diagnosing the cause of preoperative dyspnea in the patient with isolated MS. Pulmonary function and arterial blood gas testing, at rest and during exercise, may help distinguish lung disease from the pulmonary effects of heart disease. Results consistent with moderate-to-severe dysfunction at rest (*i.e.*, hypoxemia, hypercarbia, air trapping) suggest the presence of lung disease. Results equivocal at rest that worsen with exercise indicate cardiac disease, indicating that pulmonary function should be expected to improve following cardiac surgery.

The anesthetic management of patients with mitral stenosis includes any general or regional anesthetic technique fostering the appropriate hemodynamic milieu of normal-to-slower heart rates during mild afterload reduction (as necessary). Potential exacerbators of pre-existing pulmonary hypertension, such as hypoxia, hypercarbia, and acidosis, also should be identified. Routine monitoring should be adequate in asymptomatic patients with no evidence of increased pulmonary pressures, whereas invasive monitoring is warranted in patients with preoperative congestive symptoms. The latter patients may have some degree of pulmonary hypertension that should be evaluated, along with any discrepancy between the pulmonary artery diastolic pressure and the pulmonary capillary wedge pressure. Because of the gradient across the stenotic mitral valve, the wedge pressure alone is an inaccurate monitor of intravascular filling. Tachycardia will accentuate the discrepancy between the wedge pressure and the level of LV preload, producing the paradox of increasing wedge pressure in the presence of a reflex tachycardic response to hypovolemia-induced hypotension.

Prosthetic Valves

Valve prostheses may be of mechanical or organic (tissue) origin. Patients with such valves presenting for noncardiac surgery have specific preoperative requirements. Patients with mechanical prostheses require long-term anticoagulation, because the risk of thromboembolism, although greatest within the first postoperative year,[61] always is significant. Postoperative antiplatelet agents also are recommended.[62] Neither therapy precludes thromboembolic events in these patients. Although tissue valves are nonthrombogenic and so reduce the risk of such episodes, anticoagulation still is required during the first 6 to 12 postoperative weeks, as well as for perioperative treatment of chronic atrial fibrillation, intra-atrial intraoperative clot, a dilated or calcified left atrium, or for a previously documented embolic event.[63] Oral administration of anticoagulant therapy can be safely discontinued several days before surgery. If necessary, intravenous therapy can be used during the postoperative period, and oral agents can be restarted postoperatively. Patients with both types of artificial valves are at risk of endocarditis and should receive appropriate antibiotic prophylaxis.

Hemodynamically, mechanical and tissue valves are not significantly different. Since the orifice size of both is less than that of a normal valve,[63] a transvalvular gradient, although hemodynamically insignificant, will exist. A preoperative two-dimensional echocardiogram can be obtained postoperatively to assure proper prosthetic valve function.[64,65]

References

1. Skinner JF, Pearce ML: Surgical risk in the cardiac patient. J Chronic Dis 17:57, 1964
2. Goldman L, Caldera DL, Nussbaum SR et al: Multifactorial index of cardiac risk in non-cardiac surgical procedures. N Engl J Med 297: 845, 1977
3. Ross J Jr: Cardiac function and myocardial contractility: A perspective. J Am Coll Cardiol 1:52, 1983
4. Ross J Jr: After-load mismatch in aortic and mitral valve disease: Implications for surgical therapy. J Am Coll Cardiol 5:811, 1985
5. Mann T, McLaurin LP, Grossman W et al: Assessing the hemodynamic severity of acute aortic regurgitation due to infective endocarditis. N Engl J Med 293:108, 1975
6. Nishimura RA, Miller FA, Callahan MJ et al: Doppler echocardiography: Theory, instrumentation, technique and application. Mayo Clin Proc 60:321, 1985
7. Abbasi AS, Allen MW, DeCristofaro D et al: Detection and estimation of the degree of mitral regurgitation by range-gated pulsed Doppler echocardiography. Circulation 61:143, 1980
8. Pearlman AS: Assessing valvular regurgitation by pulsed Doppler echocardiography. J Cardiovasc Med 6:251, 1981
9. O'Rourke RA: Value of Doppler echocardiography for quantifying valvular stenosis or regurgitation. Circulation 78:483, 1988
10. Jaffe WM, Roche AHG, Coverdale HA et al: Clinical evaluation versus Doppler echocardiography in the qualitative assessment of valvular heart disease. Circulation 78:267, 1988
11. Braunwald E: Valvular Heart Disease. In Braunwald E: Heart Disease. Philadelphia, WB Saunders, 1988
12. Veryat C, Lessana A, Abitbol G et al: New indexes for assessing aortic regurgitation with two-dimensional Doppler echocardiographic measurements of the regurgitant aortic valvular area. Circulation 68:998, 1983
13. Masuyama T, Kodama K, Kitabatake A et al: Non-invasive evaluation of aortic regurgitation by continuous-wave Doppler echocardiography. Circulation 73:460, 1986
14. Manyari DE, Nolewajka AJ, Kostuk WJ: Quantitative assessment of aortic valvular insufficiency by radionuclide angiography. Chest 81:170, 1982
15. Hood WP, Rackley CE, Rolett EL: Wall stress in the normal and hypertrophied human left ventricle. Am J Cardiol 22:550, 1968

16. Peterson MB, Lesch M: Protein synthesis and amino acid transport in the isolated rabbit right ventricular papillary muscle. Circ Res 31:317, 1972

17. Hanrath P, Mathey DG, Siegert R et al: Left ventricular relaxation and filling pattern in different forms of left ventricular hypertrophy: An echocardiographic study. Am J Cardiol 45:15, 1980

18. Betocchi S, Bonow RO, Bacharach SL et al: Isovolumetric relaxation period in hypertrophic cardiomyopathy: Assessment by radionuclide angiography. J Am Coll Cardiol 7:74, 1986

19. Topol EJ, Traill TA, Fortuin NJ: Hypertensive hypertrophic cardiomyopathy of the elderly. N Engl J Med 312:177, 1985

20. Sanderson JE, Gibson DG, Brown DJ et al: Left ventricular relaxation and filling in hypertrophic cardiomyopathy. An echocardiographic study. Br Heart J 40:596, 1978

21. Grossman W, McLaurin P, Moos SP et al: Wall thickness and diastolic properties of the left ventricle. Circulation 49:129, 1974

22. Carroll JD, Hess OM, Hirzel HO, et al: Exercise-induced ischemia: The influence of altered relaxation on early diastolic pressures. Circulation 67:521, 1983

23. Gunther S, Grossman W: Determinants of ventricular function in pressure overload hypertrophy in man. Circulation 59:679, 1979

24. Green SJ, Pizzarello RA, Padmanabhan VT et al: Relation of angina pectoris to coronary-artery disease in aortic valve stenosis. Am J Cardiol 55:1063, 1985

25. Grayboys TB, Cohn PF: The prevalence of angina pectoris and abnormal coronary arteriograms in severe aortic valvular disease. Am Heart J 93:683, 1977

26. Hinquell L, Odoroff CL, Honig CR: Inter-capillary distance and capillary reserve in hypertrophied rat hearts beating in situ. Circ Res 41:400, 1979

27. Marcus ML: Effects of Cardiac Hypertrophy on the Coronary Circulation. In Marcus ML: The Coronary Circulation in Health and Disease. New York, McGraw-Hill, 1983

28. McDonald IG: Echocardiographic assessment of left ventricular function in aortic valve disease. Circulation 53:860, 1976

29. DeMaria AN, Bommer W, Joye J et al: Value and limitations of cross-sectional echocardiography of the aortic valve in the diagnosis and quantification of valvular aortic stenosis. Circulation 62:304, 1980.

30. Godley RW, Green D, Dillon JC et al: Reliability of two dimensional echocardiography in assessing the severity of valvular aortic stenosis. Chest 79:657, 1981

31. Weyman AE: Cross-sectional echocardiographic assessment of aortic obstruction. Acta Med Scand (Suppl 627):120, 1979

32. Currie PJ, Hagler DJ, Seward JB et al: Instantaneous pressure gradient: A simultaneous Doppler and dual catheter correlative study. J Am Coll Cardiol 7:800, 1986

33. Grossman W: Why is left ventricular diastolic pressure increased during angina pectoris? J Am Coll Cardiol 5:607, 1985

34. Otto CM, Pearlman AS, Gardner CL: Hemodynamic progression of aortic stenosis in adults assessed by Doppler echocardiography. J Am Coll Cardiol 13:545, 1989

35. Miller FA: Aortic stenosis: Most cases no longer require invasive hemodynamic study. Editorial. J Am Coll Cardiol 13:551, 1989
36. Gorlin R, Gorlin SG: Hydraulic formula of the area of stenotic mitral valve, other cardiac valves and central circulatory shunts. Am Heart J 41:1, 1951
37. Morrow AG, Roberts WC, Ross J Jr et al: Clinical staff conference. Obstruction to left ventricular outflow: Current concepts of management and operative treatment. Ann Int Med 69:1255, 1968
38. Smith N, McAnulty JH, Rahimtoola S: Severe aortic stenosis with impaired left ventricular function and clinical heart failure: Results of valve replacement. Circulation 58:255, 1978
39. O'Keefe JH Jr, Vlietstra RE, Bailey KR et al: Natural history of candidates for balloon aortic valvuloplasty. Mayo Clin Proc 62:986, 1987
40. Kay PH, Paneth M: Aortic valve replacement in the over seventy age group. J Cardiovasc Surg 22:312, 1981
41. Craver JM, Weintraub WS, Jones EL et al: Predictors of mortality, complications and length of stay in aortic valve replacement for aortic stenosis. Circ Suppl I 78:I 85, 1988
42. Magovern JA, Pennock JL, Campbell DB et al.: Aortic valve replacement and combined aortic valve replacement and coronary artery bypass grafting: Predicting high risk groups. J Am Coll Cardiol 9:38, 1987
43. Edmunds LH Jr, Stephenson LW, Edre RN et al: Open-heart surgery in octogenarians. N Engl J Med 319:131, 1988
44. Christakis GT, Weisel RD, David TE et al: Predictors of operative survival after valve replacement. Circ Suppl I 78:I 25, 1988
45. McKay RG, Safian RD, Lock JE et al.: Balloon dilatation of calcific aortic stenosis in elderly patients: Postmortem intraoperative and percutaneous valvuloplasty studies. Circulation 74: 119, 1986
46. Roth RB, Palacios IF, Block PC: Percutaneous aortic balloon valvuloplasty: Its role in the management of patients with aortic stenosis requiring major non-cardiac surgery. J Am Coll Cardiol 13:1039, 1989
47. Rappaport E: Natural history of aortic and mitral valve disease. Am J Cardiol 35:221, 1975
48. Selzer A, Cohn E: Natural history of mitral stenosis. A review. Circulation 45:878, 1975
49. Wood P: An appreciation of mitral stenosis. Br Med J 1:1051, 1954
50. Gash AK, Carabello BA, Cepin D et al: Left ventricular ejection performance and systolic muscle function in patients with mitral stenosis. Circulation 67:148, 1983
51. Heller SG, Carleton RA: Abnormal left ventricular contraction in patients with mitral stenosis. Circulation 42:1099, 1970
52. Feigenbaum H, Campbell RW, Runsch CM et al: Evaluation of the left ventricle in patients with mitral stenosis. Circulation 34:462, 1966
53. Bolen JL, Lopes MG, Harrison DC et al: Analysis of left ventricular function in response to after-load changes in patients with mitral stenosis. Circulation 52:894, 1975
54. Ahmed SS, Regan TJ, Fiore JJ et al: The state of the left ventricular myocardium in mitral stenosis. Am Heart J 94:28, 1977
55. Wroblewski E, Spann JF, Bove AA: RV performance in mitral stenosis. Am J Cardiol 47:51, 1981

56. Friedman BL, Macias DJ, Yu PN: Pulmonary function studies in patients with mitral stenosis. Am Rev Tuberc 79:265, 1959
57. Wood TE, McLeod P, Anthonisen NR et al: Mechanics of breathing in mitral stenosis. Am Rev Resp Dis 104:52, 1971
58. White HC, Butler J, Donald KW: Lung compliance in patients with mitral stenosis. Clin Sci 13: 137,1954
59. DeTroyer A, Estenne M, Yernault JC: Disturbance of respiratory muscle function in patients with mitral valve disease. Am J Med 69:867, 1980
60. Kannel WB, Seidman JM, Fercho W et al: Vital capacity and congestive heart failure: The Framingham study. Circulation 49:1160, 1974
61. Edmunds LH Jr: Thromboembolic complications of current cardiac valvular prostheses. Ann Thorac Sur 34:96, 1981
62. Shattel LFB: The prevention of prosthetic valve thromboembolism: Uses and limitations of anti-platelet drugs. Int J Cardiol 3:87, 1987
63. Braunwald E: Valvular Heart Disease. In Braunwald E: Heart Disease, p 1063. Philadelphia, WB Saunders, 1984.
64. Morris DC: Management of patients with prosthetic heart valve. Curr Probl Cardiol 7:August, 1982
65. Shapira JN, Martin RP, Fowles RE et al: Two-dimensional echocardiographic assessment of patients with bioprosthetic valve. Am J Cardiol 43:510, 1979

Paul R. Hickey
Susan Streitz

Preoperative Assessment of the Patient with Congenital Heart Disease

3

Preoperative evaluation of patients having a history of congenital heart disease (CHD) is complicated by the diversity of congenital lesions and paucity of information about cardiac risk in these patients. Numerous congenital cardiac defects of varying severity, sometimes in combination, produce complex and dynamic pathophysiologic patterns that change with growth, thereby precluding simple formulas for assessing risk. Palliative and corrective surgeries improve hemodynamic status, but rarely result in normal cardiovascular anatomy or physiology. Multiple repair procedures may be necessary for some lesions, but most procedures are poorly studied. Thus the perioperative risk factors for anesthesia and noncardiac surgery in patients with CHD can only be estimated from the natural history of the particular form of CHD and the known postoperative complications of its surgical treatment.

Extrapolation of these risk factors to noncardiac surgical patients is fraught with potential problems, now magnified by the number of CHD survivors. Each year, 8 of 1000 newborns have some form of CHD,[1] one third of these requiring catheterization or surgery within their first year.[2] Previously, only about 30% of infants with critical CHD survived their first 4 weeks;[3] now 60% or more survive the first year. Many of those who have undergone repair of their defect require subsequent anesthetics and operations during development.

SPECIFIC PROBLEMS ENCOUNTERED IN CHD

The lesions and combinations of lesions encountered in CHD patients produce only a limited set of problems that decrease cardiopulmonary reserve. Hypoxemia with cyanosis results from mixing, or inadequate pulmonary blood flow; congestive heart failure results from volume or pressure overload of the heart; pulmonary vascular obstructive disease is caused by excessive pulmonary blood flow and pressure due to shunts; dysrhythmias have both congenital and iatrogenic origins; obstruction to left heart outflow is produced by stenosis at various sites; and coronary ischemia is the result of both congenital defects and iatrogenic intrusions.

Inadequate Pulmonary Flow (Severe Hypoxemia)

After infancy, the cyanotic patient manifests special problems resulting from adaptations to chronic hypoxemia. These adaptations include polycythemia, increased blood volume and vasodilation, neovascularization, and alveolar hyperventilation with chronic respiratory alkalosis. Combined, these conditions may limit cardiac reserve and oxygen delivery during the stress of anesthetic induction and operation.[4]

Polycythemia increases the hematocrit and viscosity of the blood to dangerously high levels that may cause vascular stasis and worsen tissue hypoxia.[5] Although an increased hematocrit improves the oxygen-carrying capacity of the blood, the increased blood viscosity will decrease cardiac output when the hematocrit is greater than 60%. Patients with polycythemia and cyanosis have increased risk for renal or cerebral thrombosis, particularly if they become dehydrated.[6] Hematocrits greater than 70% appear to be associated with increased risk of cerebrovascular accidents and coagulopathies. Such patients may have a history of such accidents and some residual neurologic deficits. They should be hydrated intravenously the evening before induction of anesthesia and postoperatively until oral intake is possible. Patients whose hematocrit exceeds 60% to 70% may benefit from erythrophoresis. They also have coagulopathies, due partially to decreased levels of platelets and fibrinogen,[7] which increase their risk of excess intraoperative bleeding. Preparations should be made for intraoperative transfusion of clotting factors, if required.

Excessive Pulmonary Blood Flow

Excessive pulmonary blood flow is common in CHD and results in both cardiac and pulmonary problems. Volume overload of the ventricles always compromises cardiac reserve, independent of the presence of frank congestive heart failure (CHF). Increased pulmonary artery pressure and blood flow may limit gas exchange by several mechanisms. Compression of large bronchi by distended pulmonary vessels may obstruct the large and small airways and increase the work of breathing. The increased volume of pulmonary venous return distends the left atrium, potentially obstructing the left mainstem bronchus. Most importantly, increased pulmonary blood flow and pressure combine with elevated left atrial pressure to produce pulmonary venous congestion and increased interstitial and alveolar lung water. The resultant deterioration in lung compliance and increase in airway resistance is clinically manifest as a tachypneic, sometimes wheezing, child. Regions with atelectasis and intrapulmonary shunt will contribute to systemic arterial desaturation, even in a child with acyanotic heart disease and left-to-right shunting.

The net effects of prolonged, excessive pulmonary blood flow and pressure are hypertrophy of the medial layer of pulmonary arteries, intimal thickening and an increase in pulmonary vascular resistance, resulting in pulmonary vascular obstructive disease (PVOD).[8,9] When pulmonary vascular resistance equals or exceeds systemic vascular resistance, a left-to-right shunt will become a right-to-left shunt (Eisenmenger syndrome). These changes may occur during the first year of life in lesions such as an atrioventricular canal, or over decades, as in atrial septal defects.[10,11] Depending on the severity and duration of these changes, correction of the underlying lesion may reverse the pulmonary vascular changes to varying degrees.

Congestive Heart Failure (CHF)

The child with CHD develops CHF because of increased pressure or volume loads on the ventricles, or a combination of both. Patients compensate by well-known mechanisms. Increased catecholamine production redistributes cardiac output to favored organs, increases heart rate, decreases skin temperature, and frequently induces a catabolic nutritional state.[12] Pulmonary congestion increases the work of breathing and caloric demand while tachypnea limits intake.

Derangements vary with the severity of CHF. Evaluation of the most severe cases reveals a small child with body weight well below the third percentile for age, who is tachypneic, tachycardic, and dusky in room air. He or she may have chest wall retractions, expiratory wheezes, and diffuse rhonchi. Capillary refill may be prolonged, the extremities may be cool to the touch, and palpable hepatomegaly may be present. Preoperative chest X-ray demonstrates cardiac enlargement and increased pulmonary vascular markings with areas of atelectasis, despite hyperexpansion of the lungs. Medical management requires administration of digoxin and diuretics, which may induce a profound metabolic hypochloremic alkalosis with potassium depletion.

Other children with lesser degrees of CHF may be only mildly symptomatic, but still have substantially decreased cardiovascular reserves. The additional stress of anesthesia and surgery may produce decompensation, especially in severe cases of CHF, where compensation depends on maximal sympathetic tone. The reversibility of the ventricular dysfunction accompanying CHF in CHD is variable, but generally depends on the severity of the defect, its correctability, and the duration of ventricular dysfunction.

Dysrhythmias

Some patients with CHD have dysrhythmias of congenital or iatrogenic origin that may limit cardiovascular reserve and increase perioperative risk. Iatrogenic dysrhythmias are attributable to many sources, including anesthetic agents or chronic cardiac medications. CHD patients who may be receiving antiarrhythmic drugs or have implanted pacemakers must be evaluated for instrinsic cardiac rate and rhythm, characteristics of pacemaker function, electrolyte disorders, and current drug regimens.

Patients with congenital complete heart block usually tolerate a low heart rate for many years before pacemaker implantation is necessary. However, patients with surgically induced complete heart block require immediate temporary pacing. A permanent pacing system is needed if atrioventricular conduction has not resumed in 10 days, because it rarely returns after this time.[13] If electrocautery is to be used intraoperatively, setting the pacemaker to an asynchronous mode will protect against interference from inappropriate sensing. Pacemaker failure in CHD patients with permanent pacing systems will result in asystole. Electrocautery occasionally has caused complete pacemaker failure in congenital heart patients through burnout of the pacemaker generator unit. Thus, external pacing capabilities or pacing through a temporary wire may be emergently needed in these cases. Alternatively, the use of a bipolar cautery would not interfere with normal pacemaker function or cause damage to the pacemaker generator circuits.

OBSTRUCTION TO LEFT HEART OUTFLOW

Congenital lesions producing obstruction to outflow from the left heart include interruption of the aortic arch, coarctation of the aorta, aortic stenosis (subvalvular, valvular, or supravalvular), mitral stenosis and atresia, and hypoplastic left heart syndrome. These patients may have left ventricular hypertrophy, coronary ischemia, and limited systemic ventricular reserve. Systemic perfusion in neonates may depend on a narrowing patent ductus arteriosus, and these infants may manifest shock, metabolic acidosis, and ventricular fibrillation. Older children with less severe forms of stenosis may be asymptomatic or demonstrate dysrhythmias, syncope, fatigue, or chest pain.

Coronary Ischemia

Acquired coronary-artery disease is rare in children with CHD. However, coronary ischemia may occur with left heart outflow obstruction or anomalous coronary arteries arising from the pulmonary artery, producing coronary steal. In anomalous coronary arteries, retrograde flow into the pulmonary artery occurs through anastomotic connection with normal coronary arteries when flow is stolen from higher pressure coronary arteries originating from the aortic root. Myocardial infarctions and ventricular dysfunction can result, but may be reversible if detected and corrected early in life.

More rarely, patients may have aberrant sinusoidal coronary arteries arising directly from the right ventricular cavity. These arteries provide nutrient, antegrade (albeit slightly hypoxemic) flow into the coronary bed as long as high (systemic) pressures are maintained in the right ventricle. Any intervention that substantially decreases right ventricular intracavitary pressure results in intractable, and often fatal, coronary ischemia. When right ventricular pressure decreases, flow becomes retrograde into the right ventricular cavity, being stolen from adjacent, communicating coronary arterial beds.

More commonly, coronary ischemia has perioperative iatrogenic origins. For example, the arterial switch operation for transposition of the great arteries in small infants entails transplantation of the coronary arteries from the right to the left ventricular outflow tract. Coronary-artery stenosis and ischemia may develop intraoperatively or postoperatively. Even in patients with normal coronary arteries and dilated hearts, the stress of high afterload and tachycardia can result in coronary ischemia.

Combined Problems

The problems just described may combine in varying ways in some patients with CHD. In older patients having more complex lesions that cannot be readily corrected, ventricular function may be gradually deteriorating because of long-standing ventricular pressure or volume overload. Similarly, chronic volume loading of the heart accompanies aortic or mitral valve regurgitation and long-standing pulmonary-to-systemic arterial shunts. These patients may have only mild-to-moderate hypoxemia, despite the complete mixing due to a large shunt and excessive pulmonary blood flow. However, their near-normal levels of arterial oxygen saturation result in chronic ventricular dilatation and potential PVOD. Thus, they manifest hypoxemia and mild cyanosis, some degree of PVOD, and left ventricular dilatation with progressively decreasing ejection fractions.

Preoperative assessment of complex patients should: (1) estimate the functional limitation of CHD as an indicator of myocardial performance and reserve; (2) quantify the degree of cyanosis and magnitude of pulmonary blood flow; and, (3) evaluate pulmonary vascular resistance. For example, a patient with a long-standing Waterston shunt who is only mildly cyanotic but easily fatigued, with a heaving precordium and bounding pulses, is likely to have a high normal hematocrit with an oxygen saturation in the upper eighties. Pulmonary blood flow will be torrential, and pulmonary vascular resistance irreversibly elevated, the latter factor excluding the patient from cardiac surgical repair.

METHODS OF PREOPERATIVE ASSESSMENT

Preoperative assessment of the child with CHD includes history-taking, physical examination, electrocardiography, chest x-ray, laboratory tests, echocardiography, and cardiac catheterization. The clinical and laboratory data routinely obtained preoperatively provide important information (Table 3-1).

As many as 20% of infants with CHD will have extracardiac anomalies; 8.5% of infants with CHD will fall into a specific syndrome category.[14,15] The presence of extracardiac anomalies complicates anesthetic management and may alter risk. Infants with Down's syndrome, Treacher Collins, and Pierre–Robin may, for example, have airway abnormalities as well as CHD. Similarly, calcium and immunologic deficiencies accompany aortic arch abnormalities, and renal abnormalities occur in patients with esophageal atresia and CHD.[16]

History

A complete history should be taken, including a special review of symptoms indicative of cardiorespiratory status. Children with CHD may be asymptomatic or have signs of cyanosis or CHF. Manifestations of CHF in infants include tachypnea and dyspnea, which result in feeding difficulties and failure to thrive. Children with chronically overcirculated lungs are more susceptible to respiratory infections, the origins of which may be difficult to isolate to CHF or to infection. Older children may tire more easily than their peers or require prolonged rest periods.

TABLE 3-1.   Clinical and Laboratory Information Needed for Perioperative Assessment of Congenital Heart Diseases

History and physical examination
ECG
Chest x-ray
Complete blood count, BUN, creatinine, and electrolytes
Calcium & glucose
Two-dimensional echocardiogram and Doppler flow study
Cardiac catheterization

The presence, degree, and duration of hypoxemia are important. Cyanosis may be present at rest, or may be induced by crying and exercise. In children with severe, long-standing cyanosis, a history of hemoptysis suggests development of bronchial collaterals. Other symptoms of heart disease include squatting, palpitations, and chest pain. A history of penicillin allergy is significant, because these children will require SBE prophylaxis. A review of past and present medications should include digoxin, diuretics, beta blockers, or antiarrhythmics. Patients in the intensive care unit preoperatively may be receiving prostaglandins and inotropic agents. Patients and their parents should be questioned about prior surgery and anesthesia, particularly for details of any previous palliative or reparative cardiac procedures.

Physical Examination

The purpose of the physical examination is to characterize the disease process and to identify related problems, not to establish a specific anatomic diagnosis. First is the gross assessment of the child's well-being. Does the child appear frail and chronically ill, well-compensated, or thriving? The height and weight of the child should be compared to age-matched cohorts using standard curves. Failure to thrive usually is a sign of CHF, unless hypoxemia is severe. The values for pulse, respiratory rate, and blood pressure within the normal range for age should be known, and blood pressure in the upper and lower extremities should be measured. Blood pressure in the upper extremities of patients with aortic arch abnormalities often will be higher than pressure in the lower extremities. If the subclavian artery has been sacrificed for a classic Blalock–Taussig shunt, blood pressure in that extremity will be misleading as an estimate of central aortic pressure.

The cardiac examination should include inspection of precordial activity and auscultation of heart sounds, murmurs, and clicks. Changes in posture, respiration, or volume status will alter this examination. Patients with tetralogy of Fallot, for example, will generally have a loud systolic murmur that changes with squatting. During a *tet spell*, the murmur will be soft or nonexistent.

The patient's respiratory pattern should be assessed for signs of respiratory distress or infection and associated airway anomalies. Baseline pulmonary function should be determined to evaluate ventilatory adequacy postoperatively. Examination of the extremities provides useful information about the child's circulation. Patients with

CHF and aortic arch abnormalities may have diminished peripheral pulses, whereas those with lesions such as aortic insufficiency and patent ductus arteriosus may have bounding pulses. Peripheral edema also may be a sign of CHF. Clubbing will appear after 3 months of age in patients with cyanotic CHD. The extremities should be examined for the scars of previous incisions for venous or arterial access that may limit venous or arterial catheterization sites.

Laboratory Tests

In the absence of iron deficiency, the hematocrit is a good indicator of the degree and duration of hypoxemia. Its physiologic nadir during infancy may contribute to left-to-right shunting by decreasing relative pulmonary vascular resistance.[17] Electrolyte abnormalities may accompany CHF and forced diuresis. Children receiving diuretics may be hypokalemic. Diuresis also may lead to iatrogenic dehydration, an increase in BUN and creatinine, or hypochloremic metabolic alkalosis. Metabolic acidosis may be due to severe hypoxemia or insufficient cardiac output. Calcium and glucose also should be measured in neonates.

Chest Roentgenogram

The chest X-ray should be analyzed for heart size and position, liver site, pulmonary vascular congestion, airway compression, and areas of consolidation or atelectasis. The position of the heart relative to the viscera also should be determined. Malposition of the heart is apparent in patients with asplenia and polysplenia syndrome and is associated with complex CHD and high cardiac perioperative risk. To assess heart size accurately, the chest film should be taken with the patient in an upright position. A thymic shadow, apparent in children younger than 1 year, may complicate this assessment. A cardiothoracic ratio higher than 50% is abnormal and could indicate cardiomegaly or pericardial effusion.

Patients with tetralogy of Fallot have boot-shaped hearts, whereas the hearts of patients with total anomalous pulmonary venous return are shaped like snowmen or figures of eight. Patients with left-to-right shunt ratios greater than 2:1 will have evidence of increased pulmonary vascularity. A small pulmonary artery and pulmonary vessels that extend only to the midlung are indicative of a right-to-left shunt. The chest x-ray also may show airway compression from an anomalous vessel or evidence of an infection. Most importantly, a normal chest x-ray does not exclude the possibility of severe, complex CHD.

Electrocardiography

The electrocardiogram (ECG) rarely is diagnostic of a specific cardiac lesion, but provides useful data about heart rate and rhythm, ventricular strain, and hypertrophy. The criteria for ventricular hypertrophy will vary with age, reflecting the maturation of the cardiovascular system. The ECG should be evaluated for ventricular strain patterns (ST and T-wave changes) characteristic of excessive pressure or volume burdens on the ventricles. Evidence of myocardial ischemia also may be detected in patients with some forms of CHD (*vide supra*).

Echocardiographic and Doppler Echo Assessments

Advances in echocardiographic imaging of the heart have significantly improved the diagnosis and evaluation of CHD.[18] In some children, this noninvasive technique can replace cardiac catheterization and, in others, provide an accurate anatomic diagnosis. An echocardiogram is all that may be necessary for diagnosis of atrial septal defect, patent ductus arteriosus, or coarctation of the aorta. However, the echocardiographic and Doppler echo techniques also have limitations.

It is not always possible to visualize atrial septal defects directly, but their presence may be inferred by the presence of right ventricular volume overload and septal shift. Similarly, ventricular septal defects in the muscular septum may not be apparent on echocardiographic examination. Additionally, the anatomy of the coronary arteries, the distal pulmonary artery architecture, and the conduits between a ventricle and either great artery are poorly imaged by echocardiography, and the pressure gradients across conduits generally are not measurable by Doppler techniques. It may be difficult to obtain an adequate window for imaging in the obese patient, older child, adult, and some postoperative patients, thus limiting the accuracy of echocardiographic diagnosis relative to that in infants and small children.

The preoperative assessment of candidates for noncardiac surgery who have undergone corrective cardiac procedures benefits from echocardiographic studies of ventricular function. To determine cardiovascular reserve, echocardiographers assess left ventricular systolic performance by measuring ventricular volumes and ejection fraction, percent shortening fraction, and velocity of circumferential fiber shortening. Left ventricular volumes and ejection fraction derived from two-dimensional studies compare favorably with volumes measured at catheterization.[19] A shortening fraction of 28% to 36% is normal and is decreased in the presence of myocardial dysfunction.[20,21] Left ventricular shortening fraction indicates function in a discrete area of the ventricle. The mean velocity of circumferential fiber shortening is a better estimate of global left ventricular systolic function, but is not as widely used by echocardiographers.[22]

Echocardiographic evaluation of right ventricular (RV) function is limited by the complex geometry of the right ventricle. There are no widely accepted methods for calculating RV volume or ejection fraction. Right ventricular-systolic time intervals have been used to assess pulmonary artery diastolic pressure, but they have limited use.[23,24] They do not predict the reactivity of the pulmonary vascular bed and are most useful when it is abnormal. Catheterization studies have revealed ventricular septal defects and elevated pulmonary vascular resistance where echocardiographic RV interval studies have suggested normalcy.[25]

Doppler measurement of pressure gradients across semilunar valves and other obstructions often are accurate. Pressure gradients can be calculated by measuring the velocity of flow at the obstructed site and converting that into a gradient[26] that can be used to predict the severity of stenosis. Echo pressure gradients often may be as accurate as those obtained during cardiac catheterization, but are not always reliable.[27] Noninvasive Doppler estimates of pulmonary and systemic blood flow correlate well with measurements of these flows at the time of cardiac catheterization.[28,29] Despite the value of echocardiographic diagnosis of anatomic defects and ventricular function, however, and the accuracy of Doppler-determined pressure gradients and valvular function, cardiac catheterization remains the standard for assessment of physiologic function.

Cardiac Catheterization in CHD

Preoperative assessment of the child with CHD should include a review of the cardiac catheterization report, except for patients who have an echocardiographic diagnosis of uncomplicated atrial septal defect, patent ductus arteriosus, or coarctation of the aorta. The catheterization data must be interpreted in the context of the child's age and current clinical condition.

The physiologic data should describe the direction, magnitude, and approximate location of intracardiac shunts. The intracardiac and intravascular pressures are measured, particularly at the shunt orifices, to determine whether they are restrictive or nonrestrictive structures. Pressure gradients across sites of obstruction are influenced by blood flow at the time of measurement. Small pressure gradients measured at the time of low cardiac output may critically underestimate the severity of the obstruction. Normal intracardiac pressure and saturation values in children appear schematically in Figure 3-1.

In the absence of intracardiac pathology, there is no significant change in oxygen saturation from the *venae cavae* to the pulmonary artery. In the child with CHD, the superior vena cava gives the safest indication of true mixed-venous oxygen saturation. An oxygen saturation value higher than 80% is consistent with a high output state or partial anomalous pulmonary venous return. A saturation value below 65% suggests a low output state, aortic blood desaturation, severe anemia, or an increased metabolic rate. A 5% or higher increase in saturation from the superior vena cava to the right atrium, ventricle, or pulmonary artery suggests the presence of a left-to-right shunt.[30] This shunt would occur at the level of the right atrium in an atrial septal defect, at the ventricular level in a ventricular septal defect, and at the pulmonary artery for a patent ductus arteriosus, systemic arterial-to-pulmonary artery surgical shunt, or aortopulmonary collaterals.

The magnitude of the shunt can be calculated using the Fick equation to measure pulmonary blood flow (Qp) and systemic blood flow (Qs). A shunt is described by the ratio Qp:Qs, a term derived from measured oxygen saturations, eliminating the need to measure oxygen consumption. A Qp:Qs ratio greater than one indicates a predominant left-to-right shunt, and a Qp:Qs less than one, a right-to-left shunt.

The patient with a fully saturated aorta is assumed to have no significant right-to-left shunting and a pulmonary venous saturation equal to that in the aorta. In the presence of a right-to-left shunt, hypoxemia is documented in the aorta, and oxygen saturation is determined in the pulmonary veins, left atrium, and left ventricle. A decrease in left atrial saturation is consistent with a right-to-left shunt at the atrial level and is indicative of an atrial septal defect and right ventricular outflow tract obstruction (pulmonary atresia and intact ventricular septum), tricuspid atresia, or severe tricuspid insufficiency. It may also indicate a left superior vena cava. An increase in

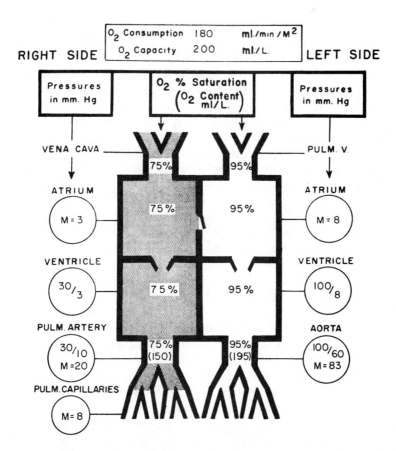

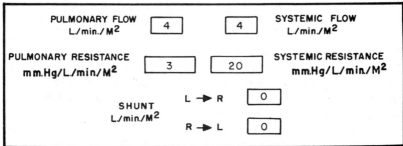

FIGURE 3-1. Normal cardiac catheterization findings in a child. Numbers in chambers are oxygen saturations(%), and numbers in parentheses are oxygen content. Pressures in chambers are shown in circles. Note probe patent foramen ovale. *(From Nadas AS, Fyler DC: Pediatric Cardiology. Philadelphia, WB Saunders, 1978)*

right atrial saturation and a concurrent decrease in left atrial saturation indicates bidirectional shunting at the atrial level (mixing). The same relationships apply at the ventricular level.

Pulmonary venous desaturation (less than 96%) implies a pulmonary source of venous admixture, and may represent significant pneumonia, atelectasis, severe congestive heart failure, or other airway disease that may substantially alter perioperative risk and, thus, anesthetic management and postoperative ventilatory requirements. Alternatively, pulmonary venous desaturation may result from heavy sedation and respiratory depression at the time of catheterization. In this case, pulmonary artery pressures may be falsely elevated and should be carefully evaluated.

The patient having a left-to-right shunt and pulmonary artery hypertension may be given 100% oxygen or a vasodilator to repeat the pressure and saturation measurements. This method will assess the reactivity of the pulmonary vascular bed and determine the contribution of ventilation-perfusion abnormalities to hypoxemia. If the pulmonary blood flow and Qp:Qs increase dramatically (with a decline in pulmonary vascular resistance) during oxygen breathing, then reactive and reversible processes, such as hypoxic pulmonary vasoconstriction from increased interstitial and alveolar lung water, contribute to elevated resistance. The relationship between indexed vascular resistance units (dynes $\cdot$ sec $\cdot$ cm^{-5}) and Wood units (mmHg $\times$ min/L/m^2) is 1 vascular resistance unit = 80 Wood units. The patient with a high fixed and unresponsive pulmonary vascular resistance and a small left-to-right shunt, despite a large shunt orifice, may have extensive pulmonary vascular damage and irreversible PVOD that will not benefit from surgical intervention.

Anatomic details are identified during cardiac catheterization by injection of radio-opaque contrast material into the chamber or vessel proximal to the obstruction or on the higher pressure side of a shunt. Angled views that may not ordinarily be used for adult catheterization provide specific information on the location and extent of a child's defect.[31,32] Ventricular function can be assessed by angiographic and physiologic recordings.

CARDIAC RISK FACTORS FOR ANESTHESIA AND SURGERY IN CHD

Cardiac risk for anesthetic and surgical procedures is largely determined by the type and severity of cardiac defect, abnormalities in the pulmonary circulation, and the presence of associated cardiac lesions.

Pulmonary vascular abnormalities vary in CHD and alter RV function and perioperative risk. Natural history studies of various lesions have identified risk factors that apply to patients whose CHD has not been surgically repaired or palliated. The surgical procedures for CHD alter these risk factors and introduce new factors in the postoperative period.

Uncorrected CHD

The perioperative risk factors for patients undergoing cardiac surgery with uncorrected CHD vary by lesion and are identified by clinical experience with surgery for CHD. Extrapolating these lesion-specific risk factors to noncardiac surgical patients is the only method available for estimating their perioperative morbidity and mortality (Table 3-2). Risk is increased with more complex and with severe lesions, with additional associated major cardiovascular anomalies, severe hypoxemia (SaO2 < 70%), with congestive heart failure and PVOD (especially with systemic or suprasystemic pulmonary hypertension), and with coronary ischemia (especially in the presence of left ventricular outflow obstruction).

Corrected or Palliated CHD

Correction of CHD by surgical or new percutaneous procedures rarely results in normal cardiovascular function, normal life expectancy, or freedom from further medical or surgical therapy, and does not decrease perioperative risk to normal levels for subsequent sur-

TABLE 3-2. General Perioperative Risk Factors for Uncorrected CHD

Severe forms of simple lesions
Complex lesions
Associated major cardiovascular lesions
Severe hypoxemia ($S_aO_2 > 70\%$)
Polycythemia (Hct > 60–65%)
Congestive heart failure
Pulmonary vascular obstructive disease
Coronary ischemia

gery. The only repairs producing normal physiology are closure of patent ductus arteriosus and atrial septal defect early in life, before the development of pulmonary vascular changes (Table 3-3).[33] Correction of all other defects results in improved hemodynamics, but not completely normal cardiovascular and pulmonary function. Some of the remaining abnormalities of function are due to irreversible disease processes, while others are iatrogenic, resulting from the procedure.

After repair of CHD, increased risk of intraoperative cardiac complications during noncardiac surgery generally is associated with the more severe or complex lesions, incomplete repairs, older age at repair, presence of PVOD, associated major cardiovascular anomalies, and age and technique of the repair. The increase in risk may be due to late dysrythmias resulting from the procedure,[34] ventricular dysfunction, residual cardiac defects and valvular dysfunction, or residual PVOD. Surgical repairs performed within the last 5 years have fewer associated problems and better outcome than those performed 10 and, especially, 20 years ago.

Preoperative evaluation of the child with a corrected congenital heart defect should include history-taking, physical examination, and ECG, echocardiographic, and catheterization data that provide infor-

TABLE 3-3. Status of Repairs for CHD Lesions

True Correction*	Correction†	Palliation‡
Patent ductus arteriosus	Coarctation of aorta	Conduits
Atrial septal defect	Transposition of great arteries	Transplantation
	Ventricular septal defect	Operations in pulmonary vascular obstructive disease
	Tetralogy of Fallot	Pulmonary atresia
	Pulmonary stenosis	Operations of the Fontan type
	Aortic stenosis	
	Atrioventricular canal repairs	

  *True Correction: Results in normal life expectancy, normal cardiovascular reserve, and freedom from further medical treatment.

  †Correction: Results in markedly prolonged life expectancy that may not be normal, with at least some limitations of cardiovascular reserve, which may require further medical, or even surgical, treatment.

  ‡Palliation: Results in prolonged life expectancy, but with definitely abnormal cardiovascular physiology, which will certainly require further medical or surgical therapy.

mation about the adequacy of repair and current cardiovascular function. All of these patients should be assumed to have residual cardiac dysfunction, even if asymptomatic. Evaluation of cardiac status and risk should apply the known medical risk factors for patients who have had repair of CHD and include the perioperative problems associated with specific lesions and types of surgical repair.

SPECIFIC LESIONS

Atrial Septal Defect

The repair of a secundum atrial septal defect (ASD) early in life results in a normal cardiovascular system. Before repair, mild to moderate left-to-right shunting occurs because of the small pressure gradient between the two atria. The shunt is generally modest, unless the ASD is extremely large. Cardiac reserve is only slightly compromised. Clinically significant PVOD does not usually develop for at least 10 or 20 years, and CHF does not develop until adult life.[35] If ASD repair is delayed until after childhood, some significant hemodynamic problems may persist. Approximately 14% of adult patients with ASD secundum will have paroxysmal supraventricular tachycardias that will persist after repair.[36]

Primum ASD with mitral valve clefts or sinus venosus-type defects accompanied by partial anomalous pulmonary venous drainage result in larger left-to-right shunts. The development of CHF and PVOD is more common, and restoration of normal function after correction less certain. Residual septal defects are uncommon after repair, but residual mitral regurgitation may occur, limiting cardiac reserve (partial atrioventricular canal).

Perioperative mortality for repair of ASD is probably less than 1%. Postoperative results are excellent for both simple ASD and for ASD with partial anomalous pulmonary venous drainage (sinus venosus defect).[37] If CHF is not significant preoperatively, postoperative cardiovascular reserve and longevity are essentially normal. Anatomic variants of simple ASD do not appreciably influence risk of intraoperative complications or postoperative morbidity.[37]

Patent Ductus Arteriosus

The large patent ductus provides a nonrestrictive left-to-right shunt between the systemic and pulmonary circulation that may cause CHF, hypoperfusion of systemic organs, and increased work of breathing, thereby limiting cardiopulmonary reserve. A smaller ductus with restrictive shunting may result in a much smaller shunt with few, if any, symptoms. PVOD develops later in life in these cases. If the patent ductus arteriosus is ligated or pharmacologically closed with indomethacin early in life, cardiopulmonary function is normal, so long as other disease processes do not supervene. During ductus ligation, there is risk of inadvertent ligation of the left pulmonary artery or the descending aorta.

The perioperative risk of ligation approaches zero in infants and children.[37] Percutaneous closure in the catheterization laboratory is now a successful and minimal-risk option to surgical closure and can be performed on an outpatient basis.[38] The mortality and morbidity of closure increase in the very young (preterm neonates) and late in childhood or in adulthood. Morbidity and mortality are higher in preterm neonates weighing less than 1500 gm, but the major risk factors are associated with incomplete development of the pulmonary and other systems. The presence of severe pulmonary vascular disease, demonstrated by bidirectional or right-to-left shunting through the ductus, contributes to risk in adults. Similarly, a repair performed after the development of severe CHF increases subsequent risk because of irreversible decreases in postoperative cardiac reserve and longevity.

Ventricular Septal Defect

Large, nonrestrictive ventricular septal defects (VSD) result in large left-to-right shunts, producing CHF and PVOD early in life (Table 3-4). Smaller defects may be better tolerated, decreasing cardiac reserve less and slowing the onset of PVOD.[39] Multiple VSDs of the muscular type represent a risk factor because of larger shunts, increased tendency to develop PVOD, and greater incidence of residual defects after surgical closure. Residual defects may result in persistent pulmonary hypertension.

After closure of VSD, depending on the severity of the lesion, the age at repair, and the events during repair, the patient may have residual left or right ventricular dysfunction, conduction defects (including heart block), residual PVOD, or residual septal defects.[40] Ventricular dysfunction may develop as a result of left-to-right shunting of blood and left ventricular volume overload. Repair of a VSD in infancy may result in good ventricular function comparable to that in normal hearts.[41] Children who have had repairs of large VSDs later

TABLE 3-4. Physiology and Risk for Ventricular Septal Defect

Physiologic Defect	Risk Factors Before Repair	Risk Factors After Repair
L–R shunting across septal defect, increased pulmonary blood flow and volume load	Multiple defects Congestive heart failure	Residual septal defect Residual pulmonary hypertension
Pulmonary hypertension and vascular disease, with large defects	Close to 0% risk for simple VSD	Ventricular dysfunction

in childhood demonstrate LV enlargement and hypertrophy, as well as depressed indices of LV function on postoperative evaluation.[42,43]

Problems with persistent pulmonary hypertension may limit exercise tolerance and reserve in some patients with preoperatively elevated pulmonary vascular resistance. Generally, the younger the child and the lower the pulmonary vascular resistance at the time of repair, the better the chance of normal pulmonary artery pressures in the late postoperative periods.[37] In a small percentage of patients, postoperative aortic regurgitation may occur after repair of subaortic VSD. Infrequent, but potential, problems following VSD repairs include subaortic obstruction resulting from patch closure of a VSD and complete heart block, requiring a pacemaker.

Perioperative mortality for repair of simple VSDs approaches zero in centers prepared for pediatric heart surgery.[37] Young age at repair is not associated with increased risk of perioperative mortality, but the presence of multiple VSDs and associated major cardiovascular anomalies is.[44] Moderately elevated pulmonary vascular resistance does not increase perioperative risk, but may affect postoperative cardiac reserve. Excessively high pulmonary vascular resistance increases perioperative risk proportionately. In one recent study,[45] patients with a pulmonary vascular resistance of > 8 Wood units/m^2, which decreased in response to a vasodilator, did not have postoperative resistance problems if the surgical repair was intact. Those in whom pulmonary vascular resistance did not decrease to < 7 in response to the vasodilator (50%) died because of resistance problems.

Patients not responding to the vasodilator who were excluded from surgery because of excessively high pulmonary vascular resistance, had progressive pulmonary vascular disease, confirming the decision not to operate.[45]

Atrioventricular Canal (Septal) Defects

Patients with atrioventricular (AV) defects have a large left-to-right shunt, high pulmonary artery pressure, a variable degree of mitral valve dysfunction, and a tendency to develop PVOD and severe CHF early in life (Table 3-5). Surgical repair is performed as early in life as possible (optimally in the first year of life), to avoid the long-term sequelae of AV defects. Reoperation for mitral valve problems often is necessary.

Perioperative risk is related to the severity of the defect (partial vs. complete canal) and its impact on mitral valve function. Risk also is related to increased pulmonary vascular resistance and the presence of associated cardiovascular anomalies. Perioperative and late mortality for complete canal defects is much higher than that for partial canal defects (*ostium primum* atrial septal defects)[46]; young age and small size at the time of repair and high pulmonary vascular resistance are the primary risk factors in complete canal defects.

Perioperative mortality approaches zero for patients with uncomplicated partial AV canal defects, despite major cardiac symptoms,

TABLE 3-5. Physiology and Risk for Atrioventricular Canal Defects

Physiology	Risk Factors Before Repair	Risk Factors After Repair
L–R shunt with pulmonary-vascular resistance governing shunt flow	Complete canals High PVR	Mitral insufficiency Pulmonary hypertension
Pulmonary hypertension and early pulmonary vascular disease	Severe mitral insufficiency	Residual septal defect
Mitral regurgitation worsens L–R shunt	Risk for repair 2%–5% (complete canals)	Ventricular dysfunction

and is approximately 5% when the defect is accompanied by significant mitral valve incompetence dysfunction.[37] Repair of a partial canal defect does not assure long-term mitral valve competence.[47]

Perioperative mortality is much higher (28%) for repair of complete AV canal defects.[48] Rates as high as 50% have been associated with increased pulmonary vascular resistance, prior palliative procedures, and associated cardiovascular defects, but not with young age at repair. Thirteen percent of those survivors required reoperation. Patients with complete canal defects also may demonstrate excessively high pulmonary vascular resistance, with complete canal defects unrelated to hemodynamic status.[49]

Mortality associated with repair has declined over the past 15 years because the severe lesions are better understood, reconstructive techniques for the mitral valve have improved, and surgical repair is provided before pulmonary vascular resistance increases. At one center, Boston Children's Hospital, perioperative mortality for complete canal repairs was 62% from 1975 to 1977, 17% from 1978 to 1980, and 5 % through the 1980s.[50*] Mitral valve abnormalities and presence of associated cardiac lesions were cited as risk factors. Kirklin and coworkers[51] reported a 2-year 2% hospital mortality rate for repair of uncomplicated complete AV canal. Ten-year survivals of 95% for repair of complete defects are projected. Greater risk is associated with major associated cardiac abnormalities. Repair in the first year of life does not presently carry increased risk and is recommended to decrease some of the associated complications and improve long-term survival.

The evaluation of these patients for anesthetic care after repair should focus on mitral valve competence and the pulmonary circulation. After early repair of complete (or partial) AV canal, children having neither mitral insufficiency nor pulmonary hypertension may have good ventricular function and cardiac reserve, while defects repaired later in childhood may have substantial amounts of ventricular dysfunction.

Aortic Stenosis

Patients with congenital aortic stenosis have decreased cardiac output, CHF, left ventricular hypertrophy, and coronary ischemia, all of which vary in severity with the type and degree of stenosis (Table

*Castenada AR: Personal communication.

3-6). Neonates with critical valvular aortic stenosis become sick shortly after delivery and are now treated using balloon valvotomy. Other forms of congenital aortic stenosis may not become apparent until later in childhood, and often require surgical treatment.

Balloon or surgical valvotomy, valve replacement, or resection of subaortic stenosis performed during childhood have high incidences of residual complications.[52] Perioperative mortality as high as 60% has been reported in neonates with critical stenosis, declining to 4% in children older than 6 months.[52] Risk factors for neonatal death included poor preoperative condition (metabolic acidosis) and coronary insufficiency. These patients have a high risk of intraoperative ventricular fibrillation. Additional risk factors include inadequate valvotomy and persistent LV failure after repair.[53] Perioperative mortality for repair of aortic valve stenosis in older infants and children has been reported to be 5%, with a reoperation rate of 23% in the first 9 years, and a sudden death rate of 3.5% in the followup period.[54]

A 30-year study of congenital aortic stenosis[52] revealed that surgical valvotomy decreased aortic valve pressure gradients, but also increased aortic regurgitation. Recurrent or residual aortic obstruction requiring reoperation occurred in 13% of long-term survivors. The incidence of late bacterial endocarditis was nearly 5%, but the incidence of cerebral emboli or third degree heart block was only 1%.

In another series of patients who had successful surgical aortic valvotomies more than 20 years ago, 36% developed recurrent obstructions requiring reoperation, and the probability of survival was 77% at 22 years after the valvotomy. Even in those patients surviving at 22 years, only 39% were free of major complications (recurrent stenosis, reoperation, or bacterial endocarditis). Many of the survivors who did not undergo reoperation had ECG abnormalities, and one

TABLE 3-6. Physiology and Risk for Aortic Stenosis

Physiology	Risk Factors Before Repair	Risk Factors After Repair
Left ventricular obstruction	Critical stenosis in neonate	Residual or recurrent aortic stenosis
Coronary ischemia	Ductal closure in neonate	Aortic insufficiency
Ventricular failure	Coronary insufficiency	Ventricular dysfunction
	Risk of repair 5% to >20% depending on age	

third had hemodynamically significant aortic stenosis or regurgitation.[55]

Percutaneous balloon valvotomy in neonates and infants for aortic valve stenosis offers good early results. The mortality rate is lower than that for surgical valvotomy, but the incidence of complications (restenosis and regurgitation) may be higher.*

Patients who have had repair of aortic stenosis are at risk for sudden death and progressive ventricular dysfunction from residual or recurrent aortic stenosis and aortic regurgitation. Aortic valve dysfunction and associated ventricular dysfunction must be considered during the preoperative evaluation for subsequent anesthetics. Although required for nearly all patients after repair of congenital heart disease, antibiotic prophylaxis is particularly important in patients with aortic valve disease because bacterial endocarditis is more common after subsequent noncardiac surgical procedures in this group.

Systemic-to-Pulmonary Artery Palliative Shunts

The Blalock–Taussig shunt has a 5% risk of perioperative mortality, and provides palliation lasting approximately 4 years if performed by 1 month of age, and longer if performed later.[56] Both the classic and modified forms of this shunt have less perioperative mortality and fewer late complications than the Waterston, Potts, and other central shunts (Table 3-7).[57] In a recent series of 143 systemic-to-pulmonary shunt procedures in infants with complex cardiac disease, overall

*Lock JE: Personal communication.

TABLE 3-7.   Physiology and Risk for Palliative Shunts

Physiology	Risk Factors Before Repair	Risk Factors After Repair
L–R shunt to provide adequate pulmonary flow for acceptable arterial saturation (75%–85%)	Severe hypoxemia (< 70%)	Severe hypoxemia Congestive heart failure
	Risk for shunt procedures 5%–16% (less for Blalock)	Pulmonary hypertension

shunt patency after 3 years was 77%, with a perioperative mortality of 12% and a late mortality of 16%. The modified Blalock–Taussig shunt hospital and mortality rates were each 5%.[58]

Central aorta pulmonary artery shunts also are effective in palliating pulmonary artery hypoplasia in small infants with complex cyanotic congenital heart disease. Neonatal perioperative mortality is 13%, and pulmonary artery distortion does not appear to be a significant complication.[59]

The late complications associated with Waterston and Potts shunts (CHF and progressive pulmonary vascular disease) increase survivors' risk for subsequent anesthesia and surgery. Patients with complex disease who have had a Blalock–Taussig shunt are more likely to have balanced pulmonary and systemic circulations. Complications in these patients during subsequent anesthesia and surgery tend to be related to the underlying cardiac lesion, not the shunt.

Coarctation of the Aorta

Coarctation of the aorta is a form of left ventricular outflow obstruction (Table 3-8). Because of the location of the obstruction, coronary ischemia usually is not a major problem until coronary artery disease complicates the existing left ventricular hypertrophy. Severe cases in neonates are life-threatening, particularly when associated with patent ductus arteriosus and intracardiac defects.

Repair of coarctation of the aorta often results in persistent sys-

TABLE 3-8. **Physiology and Risk for Coarctation of the Aorta**

Physiology	Risk Factors Before Repair	Risk Factors After Repair
Obstruction of the descending aorta in the region of the ductus arteriosus	Neonatal age group	Systemic hypertension
	Major associated cardiovascular anomalies	Restenosis Abnormal aortic valve
LV hypertrophy, aortic valve abnormalities, and upper body hypertension	Risk for repair is about 1% (higher in neonates) Paraplegia risk of 0.4% or less	

temic hypertension due to residual stenosis. Recurrent coarctation is common. Perioperative mortality due to repair is low (around 1%), but increases, particularly in neonates, when there are associated cardiac malformations.[37] The 20-year survival rate is 97% when repair is performed before age 20, and 85% when performed later. Late deaths are attributed to associated cardiovascular problems, including myocardial infarction, aortic valve disease resulting from a high incidence of coarcted bicuspid aortic valves, and aortic disease, including aneurysm formation. Hypertension also can be a late-developing complication, reportedly occurring in two thirds of patients 15 to 30 years after surgery.[60] The rates of late hypertension and survival are similar at 10 years and 15 to 30 years after repair.[33,34]

The likelihood of repeat stenosis in very young infants is high: Those having surgery during their first year have a 16% rate of reoperation within 5 years.[63] Neonates with associated major cardiovascular anomalies have a similar rate of recurrent stenosis (6%–12%), but a higher risk of perioperative (4%–13%) and late mortality (10%–16%).[64–66] The risk of postoperative paraplegia after repair of coarctation is about 0.4%,[67] and it appears to increase in patients who have not developed the collateral circulation typical of coarctation.

Perioperative assessment of any patient requiring anesthesia and surgery after repair of coarctation should focus on the possibility of systemic hypertension and its complications, as well as that of occult aortic valve disease.

CONGENITAL MITRAL VALVULAR DISEASE AND CARDIAC VALVE REPLACEMENT IN CHILDREN

The pathophysiology of congenital mitral valve disease in children is similar to that in adults with acquired mitral valve disease (Table 3-9). Congenital mitral valve disease in children is treated by reconstructive surgery, when possible. Perioperative mortality for mitral valve reconstructions for congenital mitral stenosis is high, ranging from 13% to 38%, probably because of associated abnormalities in LV development.[37] Residual mitral stenosis and incompetence usually persist postoperatively, resulting in hemodynamic impairment.

Lesions requiring valve replacement in children tend to be severe, because valvuloplasties are performed whenever possible. Because heart size increases and relative prosthetic stenosis develops during childhood growth, prosthetic valves are undesirable. Perioperative mortality and morbidity in children requiring valve replacement is significantly higher than that in adults. Among children, mor-

TABLE 3-9. Physiology and Risk Factors for Congenital Mitral Valve Disease

Physiology	Risk Factors Before Repair	Risk Factors After Repair
Annular mitral stenosis or parachute mitral valve	Age less than 2 yr	Permanent pacemaker
Obstruction to left atrial outflow	Previous cardiac operations	Bacterial endocarditis
Pulmonary hypertension	Other valve disease	Thromboembolic episodes
LV hypoplasia	Risk for valve reconstruction, 13%–38%	Anticoagulants
	Risk for valve replacement, 12%–32%	

tality is higher in patients younger than 2 years, those with previous cardiac operations, and those requiring double valve replacement.[68] Similarly, the risk of mortality or major morbidity among survivors is high.[69] Actuarial survival 5 years after surgery ranges from 70% for aortic valve replacement to 44% for mitral valve replacement. Complications include bacterial endocarditis, a major thromboembolic event, and conditions requiring permanent pacemaker replacement. In one study, mitral valve replacements in children resulted in perioperative mortality of 32%, with late deaths in 23% of survivors at a mean of 14 months.[70]

Anticoagulation therapy has been avoided in children with prosthetic heart valves because of difficulties titrating dosage and frequent accidental trauma leading to bleeding complications. Anticoagulants may be necessary to prevent thromboembolic events,[71] however, and their attendant risks must therefore be included in perioperative risk assessment of these patients.

TETRALOGY OF FALLOT AND TETRALOGY WITH PULMONARY ATRESIA

Patients with tetralogy of Fallot (TOF) have RV outflow obstruction, an aortic orifice that overrides a VSD, RV hypertension, and varying degrees of right-to-left shunting (Table 3-10). Patients undergoing

TABLE 3-10.   Physiology and Risk Factors for Tetralogy of Fallot and Tetralogy with Pulmonary Atresia

Physiology	Risk Factors Before Repair	Risk Factors After Repair
RV hypertropy	Tet spells	Residual VSD
Ventricular septal defect	Pulmonary atresia	Residual RV outflow obstruction
Overriding aorta	Severe polycythemia	Residual pulmonic insuffficiency
RV outflow obstruction (pulmonary atresia)	Risk for repair is <5% for tetrology and pulmonary atresia	Pulmonary hypertension (peripheral pulmonic stenosis)

surgery with uncorrected TOF have all the risks associated with chronic cyanosis and right-to-left intracardiac shunting. Surgical stimulation may result in a hypercyanotic "tet" spell which can be life-threatening if the lesion is severe.

Corrected TOF often is accompanied by hemodynamic abnormalities such as pulmonary insufficiency, residual VSD, RV hypertension, and dysrhythmias. Noncardiac surgical patients may require inotropic and chronotropic support in the immediate postoperative period to compensate for these conditions.[72] Patients with TOF and pulmonary atresia have significantly higher perioperative mortality (15% at 1 month after surgery) than those with uncomplicated TOF with pulmonary stenosis[73] (5% or lower, even when repair is performed in the first year of life).[37] Perioperative morbidity for both forms of lesion is higher. In a recent review of long-term valve function after total TOF repair, 78% of patients had pulmonary insufficiency, and 65% had tricuspid insufficiency.[74] This valve dysfunction often increases ventricular volume and pressure loads, causing ventricular dysfunction.

The cardiac problems expected after repair of TOF are cardiac dysrhythmias (5%) and impaired RV or LV function.[75,76] Early repair of TOF may limit ventricular dysfunction.[43] However, many of these patients have compromised hemodynamics and, thus, less reserve during subsequent anesthesia and surgery.[77] Preanesthetic evaluation of patients with corrected TOF should focus on hemodynamics and ventricular function.

Postoperative residual VSD resulting in a significant hemodynamic shunt is one risk factor for postoperative morbidity and mortality in TOF patients, with an incidence as high as 8%.[78,79] Residual RV outflow tract obstruction may occur in as many as 12% of patients, and it is not reliably detected by postoperative measurements of the RV outflow tract gradient in the intensive care unit.[79] Isolated RV outflow obstruction in small children is associated with LV dysfunction.[80] The incidence of major residual defects following TOF repair is higher in adults.[81] One long-term evaluation of repair (10 years) reported good outcome in 71%, fair outcome in 21%, and unsatisfactory outcome in 8%.

TRANSPOSITION OF THE GREAT ARTERIES

The transposition of the great arteries (TGA) results in two parallel circulations with severe cyanosis. Bidirectional shunting (mixing) is necessary to bring oxygenated blood from the pulmonary circulation to systemic circulation (Table 3-11). Interference with this shunt decreases arterial oxygenation; treatment thus relies on increasing intracardiac shunting. Patients tend to have higher than normal pulmonary blood flow and can develop PVOD when repair is delayed.

The hemodynamic effects of TGA repair depend on age at surgery and type of procedure. Atrial repair (Mustard and Senning procedures) may result in systemic ventricular dysfunction, supraven-

TABLE 3-11. Physiology and Risk Factors for Transposition of the Great Arteries

Physiology	Risk Factors Before Repair	Risk Factors After Repair
Separate, parallel circulations	Poor mixing (severe hypoxemia and acidosis)	Atrial repair
Arterial oxygenation depends on mixing	Risk of atrial repair is 5%–15% or less	Residual SVC or pulmonary venous obstruction
		Atrial dysrhythmias
RV is systemic ventricle	Risk of arterial repair is 3%–20%	Severe RV dysfunction
	High pulmonary vascular resistance (atrial repair)	Residual pulmonic stenosis

tricular tachyarrhythmias, and sinus node dysfunction, whereas arterial repair (Jatene switch procedure) has produced none of these problems and only a low incidence of supravalvular pulmonary stenosis.

Atrial Repair: The Mustard and Senning Procedures

Perioperative morbidity may not become apparent until well after atrial repair of TGA. Although most patients are in sinus rhythm immediately following the Mustard and Senning repairs, only 40% to 66% are still in sinus rhythm 7 to 10 years later,[82-85] although junctional rhythm is apparent in 53% of Mustard repairs at 20 years.[86] Atrial dysrhythmias can appear within 5 years of both repair procedures and may result in the need for a permanent pacemaker within 10 years.[87,88] The emergent use of Holter, rather than standard, ECG monitoring techniques is likely to provide a more accurate, and consequently higher, incidence of rhythmic morbidity.[89,90]

Obstruction of pulmonary and systemic venous drainage to the heart occurs both early and late postoperatively as a result of the atrial baffles used in these repairs. The incidence of superior vena cava obstruction is 5% to 10% after Mustard operations, especially when surgery is performed in infancy, but lower after the Senning procedure. Inferior vena cava obstruction appears in 1% to 2% of patients after either repair.[37] Pulmonary venous obstruction develops less often (2%–3%) than superior vena cava obstruction after both procedures but potentially has more serious hemodynamic consequences.[37]

Hemodynamic as well as electrophysiologic abnormalities occur late after atrial repairs, even in asymptomatic patients with normal routine physical examinations. In one study, only 11 of 36 asymptomatic children had normal hemodynamics 5 years after the Mustard procedure.[89] Significant RV dysfunction that adversely affects exercise capacity develops in approximately 10% of patients after either Mustard or Senning repair.[84,91] Cardiovascular response to exercise is limited after both types of repair by abnormal RV responses to abnormal factors.[92,93]

Cardiovascular status at rest may be relatively normal in patients with atrial repair of TGA. Cardiovascular response to maximal exercise may be grossly abnormal, however, with only 42% of normal mean work and 59% of normal oxygen uptake at maximal exercise,[94] due to reductions in heart rate, systemic arterial oxygen saturation, cardiac index, and stroke volume. In one study of patients with surgically corrected (atrial repairs) or congenitally corrected TGA, pulmonary and systemic ventricular ejection fraction did not increase with exercise, and ventricular volumes were markedly higher than normal to maintain cardiac index.[95] This report suggests that RV function is abnormal with or without previous surgery, and that the RV has difficulty sustaining systemic pressure loads when performing as the systemic ventricle. Increasing age further decreases RV (systemic) ejection fraction in such hearts.[96]

Late, and sometimes sudden, mortality occurs in patients apparently doing well after atrial repair of TGA. Eight to ten years after TGA repair, approximately 10% die.[87,97] Whether the cause of sudden death is due to dysrhythmias or hemodynamic complications is unknown. Patients who do well for prolonged periods after TGA repair usually have some degree of hemodynamic compromise, atrial dysrhythmia, and compromised systemic (right) ventricular function, particularly when stressed.[98,99] Nevertheless, successful pregnancy has been reported after the Mustard operation.[100] Consequently, preoperative evaluation of patients requiring anesthesia after atrial repairs of TGA should focus on dysrhythmias and reduced cardiac reserve.

Arterial Switch Operation (Jatene Repair)

In this procedure, the connections of the aorta and coronary arteries to the heart are switched with the connections of the pulmonary artery, leaving the aorta and coronary arteries connected to the left ventricle and the pulmonary artery connected to the right ventricle. This surgery is performed as early in life as possible. Five-year outcome studies indicate a functional status superior to that provided by atrial repair.

The perioperative mortality rates for neonates undergoing this procedure are as low as 5.4%.[101] These patients are all in sinus rhythm and have normal LV function 1 year or more after operation.[101,102] Left ventricular size, systolic and diastolic function, and contractility after arterial switch repair are no different from that in age-matched children.[103] Infants undergoing this procedure in their first year have normal flow velocities across the mitral valve and in the ascending aorta 2 years after surgery. Mild aortic regurgitation has been detected in only 1 of 18 patients studied in one series and 7 of 49 patients in another.[104,105] Some degree of stenosis of the pulmonary artery occurs at the site of the anastomosis,[101–105] but requires reoperation in fewer than 5% of patients.

Total Anomalous Pulmonary Venous Connection

The pathophysiology of total anomalous pulmonary venous return involves left-to-right shunting of blood and, thus, mixing of saturated pulmonary venous return and desaturated systemic venous return in the heart. There is increased pulmonary blood flow, an increased volume load on the heart, and variable degrees of cyanosis. The addition of pulmonary venous obstruction results in severe pulmonary hypertension, pulmonary edema, and low cardiac output with more severe cyanosis. The primary risk factor for repair is obstruction to pulmonary venous drainage (Table 3-12). This obstruction is characteristic of the infradiaphragmatic type of total anomalous pulmonary venous connection, which comprises approximately 20% of all cases. Other risk factors for mortality are severity of pulmonary hypertension and young age at repair. Perioperative mortality appears to be declining from approximately 20% to 11%,[106,107] but may be as high as 40% in patients with venous obstruction in whom severe cyanosis and pulmonary edema occur early. Severe cyanosis and pulmonary edema occur early and perioperative mortality is as high as 40% in patients with venous obstruction.[106,108] In one study, mortality was as low as 2.3% in 44 infants repaired at a mean age of 15 days, one half of whom had obstructed venous return.[109] This defect recurs in 10% to 20% of patients within 6 months of the initial repair, usually requiring reoperation.

Fontan Procedure

The Fontan procedure is commonly used to repair complex CHD forms having only one ventricle that can function as a pumping

TABLE 3-12. Physiology and Risk Factors for Total Anomalous Pulmonary Venous Connection

Physiology	Risk Factors Before Repair	Risk Factors After Repair
Left-to-right shunting	Congestive heart failure	Recurrent pulmonary venous obstruction
Hypoxemia	Severe hypoxemia	
Pulmonary venous obstruction and hypertension	Pulmonary venous obstruction Risk for repair is 2%–20%, depending on presence of obstructed pulmonary veins	

chamber (Table 3-13). Perioperative risk depends on the type of primary lesion and presence of associated lesions, and outcome varies widely depending on the underlying defect. Fontan originally performed his procedure in patients with tricuspid atresia, with overall perioperative mortality of 12%, and with late mortality of 6%.[110] Of 82 survivors, 94% were in New York Heart Association Functional Class I or II. Increased mortality in this series was associated with higher pulmonary vascular resistance and pulmonary artery pressures, ventricular dysfunction, structural abnormalities of the pulmonary arteries, and very young age at repair.

Recent 5-year mortality rates for the Fontan procedure in patients with tricuspid atresia are as low as 5.3%. However, some patients with tricuspid atresia do not survive to have the Fontan procedure, due to either the severity of the underlying disease or mortality during the palliative surgical procedures necessary until patients have reached the minimal acceptable age (2–4 years) for the Fontan procedure. Surgical mortalities of 17.9% for the first required palliative procedure and 17.6% for the second, death from the disease process itself, and failure to meet criteria for the Fontan procedure reduce probable 1-year survival to 64%, and 8-year survival to 55%.[111]

Mortality rates are higher for Fontan-procedure repair of other complex forms of univentricular heart: 11.7% for the double-inlet ventricle, 24% for the more complex forms of univentricular heart disease associated with polysplenia, and 65% for complex univentricular heart associated with asplenia.[112,113]

Whatever the diagnostic category, perioperative and long-term morbidity and mortality are worse when the Fontan procedure is performed in patients without optimal criteria (normal pulmonary vascu-

TABLE 3-13. Physiology and Risk Factors for Fontan Procedure

Physiology	Risk Factors Before Repair	Risk Factors After Repair
Depends on specific lesion	Severe hypoxemia (SaO$_2$ ‹ 70%)	Lack of sinus rhythm
Usually single ventricle type	High pulmonary vascular resistance	Ventricular dysfunction
Mixing physiology	Ventricular dysfunction Risk of repair is 5%–50%, depending on lesion	Hypovolemia

lar resistance, normal LV end-diastolic pressure, no pulmonary artery stenosis or distortion, and age greater than 3 to 4 years).

The Fontan procedure produces reasonably good functional results, but abnormal hemodynamics. The cardiovascular response to exercise also is abnormal. Cardiac index may be low with exercise, and mixed venous saturations decrease markedly (to 33%) to maintain oxygen consumption.[114] Studies have demonstrated high cardiac output during exercise, despite the lack of a functional RV. The mechanisms responsible for such output were abnormal increases in heart rate, ventricular end-diastolic volume, and stroke volume index.[115]

Patients having Fontan procedures who require subsequent noncardiac surgery and anesthesia have significantly limited cardiovascular reserve. Because of their particular dependence on high central venous pressures, low pulmonary vascular resistance, normal sinus rhythm, and low left atrial pressures for adequate pulmonary flow and left heart filling, any intraoperative circumstances that alter these factors will increase perioperative cardiac risk. Potential risk factors, therefore, include hypovolemia, dysrhythmias, increased intrathoracic pressure, and myocardial depression.

References

1. Hoffman JI, Christianson R: Congenital heart disease in a cohort of 19,502 births with long term followup. Am J Cardiol 42:641, 1978
2. Fyler DC: Report of the New England Regional Infant Cardiac Program. Pediatrics 65 (Suppl 2): 375, 1980
3. Nadas AS, Fyler DC: Pediatric Cardiology, 3rd ed. Philadelphia, WB Saunders, 1972
4. Theodore J, Robin ED, Burke CM, et al: Impact of profound reductions of PaO_2 on O_2 transport and utilization in congenital heart disease. Chest 293, 1985
5. Nadas AS, Fyler DC: Pediatric Cardiology. Philadelphia, WB Saunders, 1972
6. Phornphutkul C, Rosenthal A, Nadas A: Cerebrovascular accidents in infants and children with cyanotic congenital heart disease. Am J Cardiol 32:329, 1973
7. Kontras S, Sirak H, Newton W: Hematologic abnormalities in children with congenital heart disease. JAMA 195:611, 1976
8. Haworth SG: Normal pulmonary vascular development and its disturbance in congenital heart disease. In Godman MJ (ed): Paediatric Cardiology, Vol 4, p46. New York, Churchill–Livingstone, 1981
9. Rabinovitch M, Haworth SG, Castaneda AR, et al: Lung biopsy in congenital heart disease: A morphometric approach to pulmonary vascular disease. Circulation 58:1107, 1978

10. Thgien G, Maxxucco A, Grisolia EF, et al: Postoperative pathology of complete atrioventricular defects. J Thorac Cardiovasc Surg 83:891, 1982

11. Haworth SG: Pulmonary vascular disease in secundum atrial septal defect in childhood. Am J Cardiol 51:265, 1983

12. Talner NS: Heart Failure. In Adams FH and Emmanouilides GC (eds): Moss' Heart Diseases in Infants, Children and Adolescents, 3rd ed, p 708. Baltimore, Williams & Wilkins, 1983 725

13. Driscoll DJ, Gillette PC, Hallman GL, et al: Management of surgical complete A-V block in children. Am J Cardiol 43:1175, 1979

14. Levy RJ, Rosenthal A, Fyler DC, et al: Birthweight of infants with congenital heart disease. Am J Dis Child 132:249 1978

15. Greenwood R, Rosenthal A, Parisi L, et al: Extracardiac abnormalities in infants with congenital heart disease. Pediatrics 55:485, 1975

16. Greenwood RD: Cardiovascular malformations associated with extracardiac anomalies and malformation syndromes. Clin Pediatr 23:145, 1984

17. Lister G, Hellenbrand WE, Kleinman CS, et al: Physiologic effects of increasing hemoglobin concentration in left-to-right shunting in infants with ventricular septal defects. N Engl J Med 306:502, 1982

18. Sanders S: Echocardiography and related techniques in the diagnosis of congenital heart defects. Echocardiography 1:185, 1984

19. Silverman N, Ports T, Snider A, et al: Determination of left ventricular volume in children. Echocardiographic and angiographic comparisons. Circulation 62:548, 1980

20. DeMaria A, Newmann A, Lee G, et al: Alterations in ventricular mass and performance induced by exercise training in man evaluated by echocardiography. Circulation 57:237, 1978

21. Gutgesell H, Paquet M, Duff D, et al: Evaluation of left ventricular size by echocardiography. Results in normal children. Circulation 56:457, 1977

22. Gardin J, Iseri L, Elkayam U, et al: Evaluation of dilated cardiomyopathy by pulsed Doppler echocardiography. Am Heart J 106:1057, 1983

23. Hirschfeld S, Meyer R, Schwartz D, et al: The echocardiographic assessment of pulmonary artery pressure and pulmonary artery vascular resistance. Circulation 52:642, 1975

24. Riggs T, Hirschfeld S, Borkat G, et al: Assessment of the pulmonary vascular bed by echocardiographic right ventricular systolic time intervals. Circulation 57:939, 1978

25. Silverman N, Snider A, Rudolph A: Evaluation of pulmonary hypertension by M mode echocardiography in children with ventricular septal defect. Circulation 61:1125, 1980

26. Stamm R, Martin R: Quantification of pressure gradients across stenotic valves by Doppler ultrasound. J Am Coll Cardiol 2:707, 1983

27. Hatle L, Angelsen B, Tromsdale A: Noninvasive assessment of pressure drop in mitral stenosis by Doppler ultrasound. Br Heart J 40:131, 1978

28. Goldberg S, Sahn D, Allen H, et al: Evaluation of pulmonary and systemic blood flow by 2 dimensional echocardiography using fast Fourier transform spectral analysis. Am J Cardiol 50:1394, 1982

29. Sanders S, Yeager S, Williams R: Measurement of systemic and pulmonary blood flow and Qp/Qs using Doppler and two dimensional echocardiography. Am J Cardiol 51:952, 1983
30. Freed MD, Miettinen OS, Nadas, AS: Oximetric detection of intracardiac left to right shunts. British Heart J 42:690, 1979
31. Bargeron LMJR, Elliot LP, Soto B, et al: Axial cineangiography in congenital heart disease. Radiology 56:1075, 1977
32. Fellows KE, Keane JF, Freed MD, et al: Angled views in cineangiography of congenital heart disease. Radiology 56:485, 1977
33. Stark J: Do we really correct congenital heart defects? J Thorac Cardiovasc Surg 97:1, 1989
34. Vetter V, Horowitz L: Electrophysiologic residua and sequelae of surgery for congenital heart defects. Am J Cardiol 50:588, 1982
35. Haworth SG: Pulmonary vascular disease in secundum atrial septal defect in childhood. Am J Cardiol 51:265, 1983
36. Brandenburg RO Jr, Holmes DR, Brandenburg et al: Clinical follow-up study of paroxysmal supraventricular tachyarrhythmias after operative repair of a secundum type atrial septal defect in adults. Am J Cardiol 51:273, 1983
37. Kirklin JW, Barratt-Boyes BG: Cardiac Surgery, p. 463. New York, John Wiley & Sons, 1986
38. Wessel DL, Keane JF, Parness I, et al: Outpatient closure of the patent ductus arteriosus. Circulation 77:68, 1988
39. Collins G et al: Ventricular septal defect: Clinical and hemodynamic changes in the first five years of life. Am Heart J 84:695, 1972
40. Friedman WF, Heiferman MF: Clinical problems of postoperative pulmonary vascular disease. Am J Cardiol 50:631, 1982
41. Borrow KM, Keane JF, Castenada AR, et al: Systemic ventricular function in patients with tetralogy of Fallot, ventricular septal defect and transposition of the great arteries repaired during infancy. Circulation 64:878, 1981
42. Jamakani J, Graham T Jr, Canent R Jr, et al: The effect of corrective surgery on heart volume and mass in children with ventricular septal defect. Am J Cardiol 27:254, 1971
43. Cordell D, Graham T Jr, Atwood G, et al: Left heart volume characteristics following ventricular septal closure defects in infancy. Circulation 54:417, 1976
44. Rizzoli G, Blackstone EH, Kirklin JW, et al: Incremental risk factors in hospital mortality after repair of ventricular septal defect. J Thorac Cardiovasc Surg 80:494, 1980
45. Neutz JM, Ishikawa T, Clarkson PM, et al: Assessment and follow-up of patients with ventricular septal defect and elevated pulmonary vascular resistance. Am J Cardiol 63:327, 1989
46. McGrath LB, Gonzalez-Lavin L: Actuarial survival, freedom from reoperation, and other events after repair of atrioventricular septal defects. J Thorac Cardiovasc Surg 94:582, 1987
47. Stewart S, Alexson C, Manning J: Partial atrioventricular canal defect: The early and late results after operation. Ann Thorac Surg 43:527, 1987
48. Mavroudis C, Weinstein G, Turley K, et al: Surgical management of complete atrioventricular canal. J Thorac Cardiovasc Surg 83:670, 1982

49. Haworth SG: Pulmonary vascular bed in children with complete atrioventricular septal defect: Relation between structural and hemodynamic abnormalities. Am J Cardiol 57:833, 1986

50. Chin AJ, Kenae JF, Norwood WI, et al: Repair of complete common atrioventricular canal in infancy. J Thorac Cardiovasc Surg 84:437, 1982

51. Kirklin JW, Blackstone EH, Bargeron LM Jr: The repair of atrioventricular septal defects in infancy. Int J Cardiol 13:333, 1986

52. Brown JW, Stevens LS, Holly S, et al: Surgical spectrum of aortic stenosis in children: A thirty-year experience with 257 children. Ann Thorac Surg 5:393, 1988

53. Jones M, Barnhart GR, Morrow AG: Late results after operations for left ventricular outflow tract obstruction. Am J Cardiol 60:569, 1982

54. Wheller JJ et al: Results of operation for aortic valve stenosis in infants, children, and adolescents. J Thorac Cardiovasc Surg 96:474, 1988

55. Hsich K, Keane J, Nadas A, et al: Long term followup of valvotomy before 1968 for congenital aortic stenosis. Am J Cardiol 58:338, 1986

56. Stewart S, Alexson C, Manning J, et al: Long-term palliation with the classic Blalock–Taussig shunt. J Thorac Cardiovasc Surg 96:117, 1988

57. Arciniegas E, Farooki ZQ, Hakimi M et al: Classic shunting operations for congenital cyanotic heart defects. J Thorac Cardiovasc Surg 84:88, 1982

58. Wright J, Albrecht H, Beveridge T: Palliation in cyanotic congenital heart disease. Fifteen years' experience of various shunt procedures. Med J Aust 144:178, 1986

59. Barragry TP, Ring WS, Blatchford JW, et al: Central aorta-pulmonary artery shunts in neonates with complex cyanotic congenital heart disease. J Thorac Cardiovasc Surg 93:767, 1987

60. Presbitero P, Demarie D, Villani M, et al: Long term results (15–30 years) of surgical repair of aortic coarctation. Br Heart J 57:462, 1987

61. Clarkson PM, Nicholson MR, Barratt Boyes BG, et al: Results after repair of coarctation of the aorta beyond infancy: A 10 to 28 year follow-up with particular reference to late systemic hypertension. Am J Cardiol 51:1481, 1983

62. Katz G, Uretzky G, Beer G, et al: Long-term results of surgical repair of coarctation of the aorta—evaluation by exercise tests. Cardiology 74:465, 1987

63. Beekman RH, Rocchini AP, Behrendt DM, et al: Long-term outcome after repair of coarctation in infancy: Subclavian angioplasty does not reduce the need for reoperation. J Am Coll Cardiol 8:1406, 1986

64. Kopf GS, Hellenbrand W, Kleinman C, et al: Repair of aortic coarctation in the first three months of life: Immediate and long-term results. Ann Thorac Surg 41:425, 1986

65. Goldman S, Hernandez J, Pappas G: Results of surgical treatment of coarctation of the aorta in the critically ill neonate. Including the influence of pulmonary artery banding. J Thorac Cardiovasc Surg 91:732, 1986

66. Nair, UR, Jones O, Walker DR: Surgical management of severe coarctation of the aorta in the first month of life. J Thorac Cardiovasc Surg 86:587, 1983

67. Brewer LA, Fosburg, RA, Mulder GA, et al: Spinal cord complications following surgery for coarctation of the aorta. J Thorac Cardiovasc Surg 64:368, 1972
68. Robbins RC, Bowman FO, Malm JR: Cardiac valve replacement in children: A twenty-year series. Ann Thorac Surg 45:56, 1988
69. Williams WG et al: Experience with aortic and mitral valve replacement in children. J Thorac Cardiovasc Surg 81:326, 1981
70. Zweng TN, Bluett MK, Mosca R, et al: Mitral valve replacement in the first 5 years of life. Ann Thorac Surg 47:720, 1989
71. Sade RM, Crawford FA Jr, Fyfe DA, et al. Valve prostheses in children: A reassessment of anticoagulation. J Thorac Cardiovasc Surg 95:553, 1988
72. Berner M, Oberhnsli I, Rouge JC, et al: Chronotropic and inotropic supports are both required to increase cardiac output early after corrective operations for tetralogy of Fallot. J Thorac Cardiovasc Surg 97:297, 1989
73. Kirklin JW, Blackstone EH, Shimazaki Y, et al: Survival, functional status and reoperations after repair of tetralogy of Fallot with pulmonary atresia. J Thorac Cardiovasc Surg 96:102, 198
74. Zahka K, Horneffer P, Rowe S, et al: Long term valvular function after total repair of Tetralogy of Fallot. Relation to ventricular arrhythmias. Circulation 78 suppl III:14, 1988
75. Lawrence A, Berger HJ, Johnston DE, et al: Radionuclide assessment of right and left exercise reserve after total correction of Tetralogy of Fallot. Am J Cardiol 45:1013, 1980
76. Katz, NM, Blackstone EH, Kirklin JW, et al: Late survival and symptoms after repair of tetralogy of Fallot. Circulation 65:403, 1982
77. Calza G, Panizzon G, Rovida S, et al: Incidence of residual defects determining the clinical outcome after correction of tetralogy of Fallot: Postoperative late follow-up. Ann Thorac Surg 47:428, 1989
78. Rocchini AP, Keane JF, Freed MD, et al. Left ventricular function following attempted surgical repair of tetralogy of Fallot. Circulation 57:798, 1978
79. Lang P, Chipman CW, Siden H, et al: Early assessment of hemodynamic status after repair of tetralogy of Fallot. Am J Cardiol 50:795, 1982
80. Sholler GF, Colan SD, Sanders SP: Effect of isolated right ventricular outflow obstruction on left ventricular function in infants. Am J Cardiol 62:778, 1988
81. Presbitero P, Demarie D, Aruta E, et al: Results of total correction of tetralogy of Fallot performed in adults. Ann Thorac Surg 46:297, 1988
82. Clarkson P, Barratt-Boyes B, Neutze J: Late dysrhythmias and disturbances of conduction following Mustard operation for complete transposition of the great arteries. Circulation 53:519, 1976
83. Flinn CJ, Wolff GS, Dick M(II), et al: Cardiac rhythm after the Mustard operation for complete transposition of the great arteries. N Engl J Med 310:1635, 1984
84. Deanfield J, Camm J, Macartney F, et al: Arrythmia and late mortality after Mustard and Senning operation for transposition of the great arteries. J Thorac Cardiovasc Surg 96:569, 1988

85. Bink-Boelkens MTE, Bergstra A, Cromme-Dijkhuis AH, et al: The asymptomatic child a long time after the Mustard operation for transposition of the great arteries. Ann Thorac Surg 47:45, 1989
86. Williams WG, Trusler GA, Kirklin JW, et al: Early and late results of a protocol for simple transposition leading to an atrial switch (Mustard) repair. J Thorac Cardiovasc Surg 95:717, 1988
87. Turley K, Hanley FL, Verrier ED, et al: The Mustard procedure in infants (less than 100 days): Ten-year follow-up. J Thorac Cardiovasc Surg 96:849, 1988
88. Flinn CJ, Wolff GS, Dick M, et al: Cardiac rhythm after the Mustard operation for complete transposition of the great arteries. N Engl J Med 310:1625, 1984
89. Bender H Jr, Graham T Jr, Boncek R, et al: Comparative operative results of the Senning and Mustard operation for transposition of the great arteries. Circulation 61 suppl II:2, 1980
90. Martin T, Smith L, Hernandez A, et al: Dysrhythmias following Senning operation for dextro-transposition of the great arteries. J Thorac Cardiovasc Surg 64:878, 1983
91. Kato H, Nakano S, Matsuda H, et al: Right ventricular myocardial function after atrial switch operation for transposition of the great arteries. Am J Cardiol 63:226, 1989
92. Benson LN, Bonet J, McLaughlin P, et al: Assessment of right ventricular function during supine bicycle exercise after Mustard's operation. J Thorac Cardiovasc Surg 65, 1052, 1982
93. Bender HW Jr, Stewart JR, Merrill WH, et al: Ten years' experience with the Senning operation for transposition of the great arteries: Physiological results and late follow-up. Ann Thorac Surg 47:218, 1989
94. Ensing GJ, Heise CT, Driscoll DJ: Cardiovascular response to exercise after the Mustard operation for simple and complex transposition of the great arteries. Am J Cardiol 62:617, 1988
95. Peterson RJ, Franch RH, Fajman WA: Comparison of cardiac function in surgically and congenitally corrected transposition of the great arteries. J Thorac Cardiovasc Surg 96:227, 1988
96. Graham TP, Parrish MD, Boucek RJ, et al: Assessment of ventricular size and function in congenitally corrected transposition of the great arteries. Am J Cardiol 51:244, 1983
97. Turina, M et al: Long-term outlook after atrial correction of transposition of great arteries. J Thorac Cardiovasc Surg 95:828, 1988
98. Graham T Jr, Atwood G, Borecek R Jr, et al: Abnormalities of right ventricular function following Mustard's operation for transposition of the great arteries. Circulation 52:678, 1975
99. Jarmakani J, Canent R: Preoperative and postoperative right ventricular function in children with transposition of the great arteries. Circulation 49 suppl II:II39, 1974
100. Neukermans K, Sullivan TJ, Pitlick PT: Successful pregnancy after the Mustard operation for transposition of the great arteries. Am J Cardiol 62:838, 1988
101. Planche C, Bruniaux J, Lacour-Gayet F, et al: Switch operation for transposition of the great arteries in neonates: A study of 120 patients. J Thorac Cardiovasc Surg 96:354, 1988

102. Idriss FS, Ilbawi MN, DeLeon SY: Transposition of the great arteries with intact ventricular septum. J Thorac Cardiovasc Surg 95:255, 1988

103. Colan SD, Trowitzsch E, Wernovsky G, et al: Myocardial performance after arterial switch operation for transposition of the great arteries with intact ventricular septum. Circulation 78:132, 1988

104. Wernovsky G, Hougen TJ, Walsh EP, et al: Midterm results after the arterial switch operation for transposition of the great arteries with intact ventricular septum: Clinical hemodynamic, echocardiographic, and electrophysiologic data. Circulation 77:1333, 1988

105. Gibbs JL, Qureshi SA, Martin R, et al: Neonatal anatomical correction of transposition of the great arteries: Non-invasive assessment of haemodynamic function up to four years after operation. Br Heart J 60:66, 1988

106. Oelert H, Schafers HJ, Stegmann T, et al: Complete correction of total anomalous pulmonary venous drainage: Experience with 53 patients. Ann Thorac Surg 41:392, 1986

107. Lamb RK, Qureshi SA, Wilkinson JL, et al: Total anomalous pulmonary venous drainage: Seventeen year experience. J Thorac Cardiovasc Surg 96:368, 1988

108. Bove EL, de Laval MR, Taylor JFN, et al: Infradiaphragmatic total anomalous pulmonary venous drainage. Ann Thorac Surg 31:544, 1981

109. Sano S, Brawn WJ, Mee RBB: Total anomalous pulmonary venous drainage. J Thorac Cardiovasc Surg 97:886, 1989

110: Fontan F, Deville C, Quaegebeur J, et al: Repair of tricuspid atresia in 100 patients. J Thorac Cardiovasc Surg 85:647, 1983

111. Tam CKH, Lightfoot NE, Finlay, et al: Course of tricuspid atresia in the Fontan era. Am J Cardiol 63:589, 1989

112. Humes RA, Porter CJ, Mair DD, et al: Intermediate follow-up and predicted survival after the modified Fontan procedure for tricuspid atresia and double-inlet ventricle. Circulation 76(Pt 2):III67, 1988

113. Humes RA, Feldt RH, Coburn PJ, et al: The modified Fontan operation for asplenia and polysplenia syndromes. J Thorac Cardiovasc Surg 96:212, 1988

114. Shachar GB, Fuhrman BP, Wany Y, et al: Rest and exercise hemodynamics after the Fontan procedure. Circulation 65:1043, 1982

115. Peterson RJ, Franch RH, Fajman WA, et al: Noninvasive determination of exercise cardiac function following Fontan operation. J Thorac Cardiovasc Surg 88:263, 1984

Philip G. Boysen

Preoperative Assessment of the Patient Undergoing Noncardiac Thoracic Surgery

4

NONCARDIAC THORACIC SURGERY

The decision to perform a thoracotomy to resection lung tissue is a frequent by-product of the presence of lung cancer. Most patients with lung cancer also have chronic obstructive pulmonary disease (COPD) resulting from longterm tobacco use. Surgical resection of the cancer is their only hope for cure. Resection of a cancerous lung, however, often requires removal of functional (albeit abnormal) lung tissue in patients in whom the amount of resectable lung tissue is limited due to COPD depletion of pulmonary reserve. Moreover, the removal of a critical mass of tissue results in pulmonary hypertension and *cor pulmonale*, even when lung function is normal. Thus, the compromised patient is at greater risk of permanent pulmonary impairment after surgical resection. Candidates for this procedure must be evaluated for: (1) resectability, to determine whether surgical resection for cure is possible; and (2) operability, to lessen morbidity and mortality. Resectability can be verified by anatomical investigation excluding local invasion, distant metastases, and the systemic or hormonal disease that often accompanies intrapulmonary lesions. Operability can be assessed physiologically by evaluating the baseline pulmonary function, the diseased lung's contribution to overall function (split-function studies), pulmonary vascular status, and exercise protocols.

The surgeon still must examine the open thorax to determine the extent of resection necessary to remove diseased cancerous tissue. Typically, a stepwise approach to thoracotomy is taken. After fiberoptic bronchoscopy is used to biopsy suspicious areas, a limited thoracotomy or mediastinoscopy is performed (depending on whether the lesion is leftsided or rightsided), with appropriate biopsies. If gross and histopathological examinations do not preclude resection, a full thoracotomy is possible. At the University of Florida, we prefer to evaluate all patients for pneumonectomy, being aware that lobectomy or wedge resection may then be adequate (Table 4-1). Physiologic evaluation begins with an assessment of baseline pulmonary function at rest. The standard test battery includes spirometry before and after administration of a nebulized bronchodilator, determination and compartmentalization of lung volume, and measurement of the diffusing capacity for carbon monoxide (D_{CO}).

Baseline Pulmonary Function Testing

To test baseline pulmonary function, we initially obtain three spirograms, administer a bronchodilator, then repeat three spirograms. After inspecting the spirometric tracing to ensure maximal and reproducible effort, we select the best attempt of the six tracings and, from that, calculate the forced vital capacity (FVC), the forced expiratory volume at 1 second (FEV_1), the FEV_1/FVC ratio, and midflow values.

TABLE 4-1.

Physiologic System	Manifestation
Hormonal	Adrenocortical hyperfunction
	Inappropriate secretion of antidiuretic hormone
	Estrogen secretion
	Carcinoid syndrome
	Hypercalcemia
Neuromyopathic	Cortical cerebellar degeneration
	Peripheral neuropathy or myopathy
	Subacute spinocerebellar degeneration

The latter can be expressed as the maximum expiratory flow rate (MEFR) or the forced expiratory flow between 25% and 75% of the exhaled vital capacity (FEF_{25-75}) (Fig. 4-1). We also measure the maximal voluntary ventilation (MVV), rather than estimating it, by multiplying the FEV_1 by 38.5. (We have found that a single burstlike effort is possible, while sustained movement of gas is not, particularly in the more compromised patient.) Finally, we analyze arterial blood gases: Carbon dioxide retention with both lungs intact indicates chronic respiratory failure and precludes resection of even small amounts of lung tissue; chronic hypoxia usually is accompanied by a sustained increase in pulmonary vascular resistance and poor functional status.

Appropriate baseline spirometric values, lung volume data, and diffusing capacity measurements have been standardized as absolute values and as percentages of predicted lung function, using reported data from large groups of normal individuals. The current criteria for baseline function are presented in Table 4-2. The predictive value of the FVC and the MVV measurements (known then as the maximal breathing capacity) was established in an era when most pulmonary resectional surgery was performed in tubercular patients. The MVV value consistently correlates with postoperative morbidity and mortality.[1-4] The initial FVC values were confirmed by Mittman,[5] who also identified increased morbidity and mortality in patients with

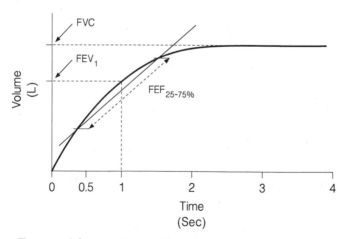

FIGURE 4-1. Idealized spirometric tracing and derived data.

TABLE 4-2. Pulmonary Function Criteria and Increased Risk

Indicator	Absolute Value Indicating Increased Risk	% Normal Value = Increased Risk
FVC	2.0 L[1]	70%[5]
	1.7 L[20]	< 70%
FEV$_1$	1.2 L[20]	
	< 2.0 L[6]	< 50%
	< 2.0 L[7]	< 50%
FEV$_1$/FVC		35%[20]
		50%[6]
MEFR	200 L/min[31]	
FEF 25–75	1.6 L/min[7]	
RV	RV/TLC	≥ 50%
D$_{CO}$(D$_{L_{CO}}$)		≤ 50%
MVV	45 L/min[1,20]	50%[1,5,10]
		55%[7]

See references 1, 5, 6, 7, 9, 10, 20, 31, 43.

lung hyperinflation and gas trapping, and correlated electrocardiographic (ECG) abnormalities to eventual pulmonary complications. Boushy[6] then established an absolute value of less than 2 L for the FEV$_1$, which was confirmed by Miller and colleagues.[7] Both Bouchy and Miller also confirmed that other indices of airflow obstruction, such as the FEV$_1$/FVC ratio and the FEF$_{25-75}$, reliably indicated postoperative functions. Lockwood[2] confirmed the overall predictive value of baseline pulmonary testing by establishing many of these same variables in a large population. In summary, determining risk and predicting postoperative status[8–10] for candidates for lung resection begins with measuring baseline pulmonary function. Failure to meet the criteria provided in Table 4-2 indicates increased risk. Patients so identified must then undergo split lung-function testing with either bronchospirometry or radionuclide scanning.

Split Function Studies

Bronchospirometry. With baseline data available for both lungs, the clinician can determine whether the removal of one lung will result in lung function adequate for survival. The first and most direct method for estimating postoperative function is bronchospirometry. The awake, supine patient is given a local anesthetic, and the trachea is intubated with a double-lumen tube. Inflation of the tracheal and endobronchial cuff isolates gas flow from the right and left lungs. Each lumen also is connected to a separate spirometer. The patient is asked to demonstrate vital capacity, during which the volume of gas from each lung and the contribution of each lung to total exhaled gas volume, can be determined. An FEV_{ppo} of 1 L is required to proceed with pneumonectomy. The predicted level of postoperative function is 800 ml, because this is the FEV_1 at which carbon dioxide retention naturally occurs in chronic lung disease.[8–10] Very small individuals and women may be exceptions. Gass and Olsen[11] suggested considering the predicted postpneumonectomy FEV_1 as a percentage of normal. Neuhas and Cherniack[12] performed these split-function studies and found that preoperative results reliably predicted postoperative function. Flow resistance data are deceiving, because resistance is due to the narrowness of the lumina, rather than the patient's own airway. Thus, FEV_1 and MVV results are unreliable; these values tend to decrease by the same fraction as the FVC.

Radiospirometry. Radiospirometry is less invasive than bronchospirometry and also provides split-function data that are reliably predictive of postoperative lung function.[13] [133]Xe is injected or inhaled, then a gamma camera is used to count the distribution of isotopes in each lung to evaluate individual function.

Perfusion Lung Scanning. Lung imaging using technetium-99m is another radionuclide study technique recently tested.[14] [99m]Tc is a less expensive, more stable isotope than [133]Xe. Although tested patients often have ventilation or perfusion abnormalities, the ventilation-to-perfusion ratio for each lung is the same.

Lateral Position Test. A fourth split-function technique, the lateral position test,[15] attempts to quantify differential lung function. Its predictive value for postpneumonectomy function has been confirmed in high-risk patients,[16] and it correlates well with radionuclide ventilation or perfusion scanning.[17] However, repeated testing of healthy nonsmokers[18] and of subjects with $FEV_1 < 2$ L[19] produces extremely variable results, indicating that the data obtained are not reliable. Thus, although easy to perform (requiring only a spirometer), this test is not widely used.

A postpneumonectomy FEV_1 is predicted using the equation:

$FEV_{ppo} = FEV_1 \times \%$ perfusion or ventilation to uninvolved lung.

If V/Q scanning indicates that a lobectomy is adequate treatment, postoperative lung function can be predicted by a second equation:

$$\text{Functional loss} = \frac{FEV_1 \times \text{functional lobes to resect}}{\# \text{segments both lungs}}$$

This scanning appears reliably predictive in pneumonectomy patients[8] and correlates with postoperative mortality in lung resection patients.[9,20]

Once split-function data are acquired, it becomes possible to determine resectability and operability. For example, $FEV_{1ppo}/FEV\text{-}N$ ratio exceeding 40% in candidates for pneumonectomy indicates a satisfactory outcome, whereas a ratio less than 30% denotes inoperability.[9]

Vascular Catheterization Studies

Pulmonary-artery hypertension often accompanies inadequate pulmonary reserve in chronic obstructive pulmonary disease (COPD) and postpneumonectomy patients,[21] resulting in decreased cardiac output, decreased cross-sectional area of the pulmonary vascular bed, and reduced exercise capacity. Resection of lung tissue may actually produce respiratory dysfunction by causing hemodynamic changes (pulmonary vascular hypertension, arterial oxygen desaturation, reduced exercise capacity, and cor pulmonale). Vascular catheterization studies were developed to estimate the postoperative effects of a pneumonectomy during a temporary and reversible alteration of flow.

Using fluoroscopy, a balloon-tipped catheter is placed into position to achieve temporary unilateral pulmonary artery occlusion of the involved lung. When the balloon is inflated, flow to the lung is temporarily occluded and proximal pulmonary artery pressure (PAP) can be measured and correlated with arterial oxygen saturation. Because ventilation rapidly shifts away from the lung with no blood flow, ventilatory data also can be accumulated. If normal data are observed at rest, low levels of exercise can be established with the patient supine, using a bicycle ergometer. Increased PAP or decreased arterial oxygen saturation (SaO_2) during exercise indicates inoperability.[21-24] Generally, a PAP exceeding 35 mm Hg, or SaO_2 less 80% (*i.e.*, $PaO_2 < 45$ mm Hg), either at rest or during exercise, precludes a pneumonectomy.

Although results are reproducible, temporary unilateral pulmonary artery occlusion is not easy to perform and requires significant expertise, specialized equipment, and much time. Also, it is invasive and risky. Fee and colleagues[25] attempted to obtain similar information using a balloon-tipped, flow-directed pulmonary artery catheter to measure PAP and thermal dilution cardiac output during treadmill exercise. Of 30 patients who underwent surgery after testing (10 open biopsies, 2 segmentectomies, 11 lobectomies, 7 pneumonectomies), 18 patients who survived had met preoperative spirometric and pulmonary vascular resistance criteria (PVR $<$ 190 dynes·sec·cm^{-5} during exercise. Five other patients who met spirometric criteria, but had elevated PVR, died. Fee and colleagues concluded that patients with elevated PVR do not tolerate lung resection, even if only small amounts of tissue are removed. The invasive nature and difficulty of performing an exercise study after pulmonary artery catheterization has limited the use of their technique.

Exercise Studies

Exercise tolerance provides information on cardiac, pulmonary, muscular, and cellular performance. Exercise protocols and patient selection criteria have so varied among studies, however, that conclusive use of this testing technique is not yet possible.

For example, Reichel[26] retrospectively studied 31 patients who underwent an incremental, graded treadmill exercise-tolerance test, applying protocols similar to those used by cardiologists. No patient who completed the six stages of testing suffered postpneumonectomy complications, whereas 57% of those who could not complete the test had complications. However, the 31 exercised patients were selected from a potential group of 75, and the selection criteria were unknown, making it difficult to apply these results to clinical practice.

Coleman[27] evaluated 54 consecutive patients prior to lung resection by measuring pulmonary function, dyspnea after a two-flight stair climb, and oxygen consumption during a multistage bicycle ergometer test. No relationship was found between maximal oxygen consumption ($\dot{V}O_{2max}$) and the development of postoperative pulmonary complications, but the cardiopulmonary complications were not isolated in the data analysis. In contrast, Eugene and colleagues[28] found a relationship between the $\dot{V}O_{2max}$ and postoperative mortality in 19 patients evaluated by bicycle ergometry. A $\dot{V}O_{2max}$ less than 1 L per minute resulted in 75% mortality and no deaths occurred when this value exceeded 1 L per minute.

In a study of cardiopulmonary complications in 22 operative pa-

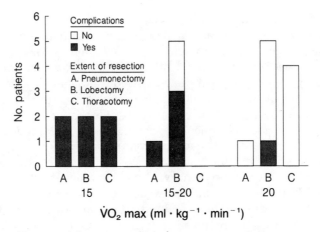

FIGURE 4-2. Preoperative $\dot{V}O_{2max}$ during exercise and the extent of resection predict postoperative complications.

tients, Smith[29] evaluated pulmonary function, radionuclide lung scans, and measured $\dot{V}O_{2max}$ during bicycle ergometry. Complications included respiratory failure, myocardial infarction, cardiac dysrhythmias, pneumonia, atelectasis, pulmonary embolism, and death in the first 30 days after surgery. Fourteen of 22 patients were identified as high-risk, based on pulmonary function data. Six patients in the high-risk group had a $\dot{V}O_{2max}$ less than 15 ml/kg per minute and postoperative cardiopulmonary complications. A $\dot{V}O_{2max}$ greater than, or equal to, 15 to 20 ml/kg per minute reduced the incidence of complications to 10% to 60%.

On the other hand, our recently collected data from 14 high-risk patients (FEV$_1$ < 2 L) during treadmill exercise revealed no difference in $\dot{V}O_{2max}$ between 5 patients who had no complications and 9 who did. Similarly, Markos and coworkers[9] found no correlation between $\dot{V}O_{2max}$ and the incidence of postoperative complications in 55 consecutive patients evaluated by bicycle ergometry. They did, however, correlate a 2% or greater increase in SaO_2 during exercise with a poor prognosis.

One explanation for the wide variability in exercise test results may be that subtle and unappreciated changes that occur in hemodynamic function are being uncovered. For example, $\dot{V}O_{2max}$ decreases in the presence of both cardiac and pulmonary dysfunction. With cardiac disorders, the arterial PaO_2 remains the same or increases, and the ratio of dead space (Vd) to tidal volume (Vt) decreases, whereas with ventilatory impairment, PaO_2 often declines, $PaCO_2$ may increase, and Vd/Vt is unchanged. Finally, in pulmonary disease, minute ventilation ($\dot{V}_E$) approaches the MVV (80%–100%) as the patient nears $\dot{V}O_{2max}$.

It is not yet clear if all preoperative patients should be studied, or only those at increased risk according to pulmonary function criteria.[29] Maximal exercise performance may not be necessary but, if it is, various measurements (maximal heart rate, maximal oxygen consumption, anaerobic threshold) have been suggested. Exclusion criteria for surgery have not been established.

Nevertheless, the following guidelines seem reasonable. First, a 3% decrease from baseline in SaO_2 during exercise suggests severe pulmonary disease with impaired gas exchange or pulmonary vascular disease, both of which correlate with a poor prognosis. If a patient cannot exercise to $\dot{V}O_{2max}$ because of dyspnea, or if the maximal $\dot{V}_E$ is more than 50% of the MVV, pulmonary (not cardiac) disease is the predominant limiting factor. Although these results probably indicate a poor prognosis (for both morbidity and mortality), they cannot be used to exclude surgical candidates at present.

Anesthetic Management

There currently are no data defining whether a particular intraoperative anesthetic technique improves outcome, in part because anesthetic management techniques continually evolve to facilitate surgical procedures. The availability of potent, rapid-onset, short-duration narcotics have made bronchoscopy and mediastinoscopy easier to manage. Although these are relatively minor procedures, they involve short periods of intense stimulation followed by brief respites from all stimulation.

The administration of a narcotic during induction of anesthesia for thoracotomy has become the preferred technique. A double-lumen tube is now routinely used. The residual effects of narcotic induction facilitate the administration of one-lung anesthesia, and allow the use of high inspired oxygen concentration, if necessary, without the addition of nitrous oxide.

During emergence from anesthesia, and in the immediate postoperative period, the use of epidural or intrathecal opiates is now routine. We use these pain management techniques in all thoracotomy patients. The result is a quiet, pain-free, and relatively comfortable patient with normal breathing patterns and the ability to sustain maximal inspiration on command and to cooperate with respiratory therapy maneuvers. Although opiate pain management risks depression of postoperative respiratory function, it may be difficult for investigators to exclude patients from epidural or intrathecal pain management measures.

Postoperative mortality and postresectional pulmonary function can be reliably predicted using various techniques. The incidence of postoperative morbidity is more difficult to determine. Invasive assessment of hemodynamic variables markedly improves our ability to indentify patients at high risk for both morbidity and mortality, but involves greater difficulty and greater risk. Exercise studies using noninvasive measurement techniques may improve patient selection and prediction of complications with less risk to the patient.

Until we have an alternative to surgery for the patient with lung cancer, we must continue to improve our techniques of preoperative assessment to improve patient survival.

NONTHORACIC SURGERY

The criteria for predetermining postoperative guidelines to asses morbidity and mortality in nonthoracic surgical patients are not as firm as those for intrathoracic resectional lung surgery. However, postoperative outcome is projected by measuring or determining preoperative lung function using the same pulmonary function tests and arterial blood-gas analyses.

Preoperative assessment of the nonthoracic surgical candidate should focus on: (1) identifying the patient with chronic airway obstruction; (2) possible preoperative therapy to modify risk; and (3) surgical incision site.[24,30] Stein and Stein and Cassara noted a 60% complication rate in compromised patients who did not receive a preoperative bronchodilator, antibiotic therapy, and chest physiotherapy, compared with a 22% rate in patients treated preoperatively.[24,30]

Most of the pulmonary function data (FEV_1, FEV_1/FVC, FEF_{25-75}, MEFR, MVV) help to identify the presence of chronic obstructive lung disease in nonthoracic patients. The changes in postoperative pulmonary function, even if preoperative pulmonary function is normal, are characteristic of a restrictive ventilatory defect. Lung volumes are decreased, and the FVC can be reduced by as much as 50% on the first postoperative day after an upper abdominal operation. The pattern of change of lung volumes usually suggests an *extrinsic* restrictive defect, since functional residual capacity (FRC) and total lung capacity (TLC) usually decrease disproportionately to the residual volume (RV). The worst effects are apparent on the first postoperative day, with recovery of 80% of function by the third postoperative day. Full recovery may take as long as 2 to 3 weeks (Fig. 4-3).

It seems likely that a superimposed but transient restrictive ventilatory defect, common with upper abdominal surgery, may increase morbidity and mortality. In a compromised patient like the COPD patient, the combined derangement in function may overwhelm the ability to maintain ventilation. Other underlying problems, such as obesity, abdominal distension, skeletal abnormalities, and interstitial lung disease, although less common, also may restrict ventilation.

Reducing the risks associated with nonthoracic surgery relies on therapeutic intervention: preoperative therapy, to maximally improve baseline pulmonary function, and postoperative therapy to reverse postoperative physiologic changes. The preoperative bronchopulmonary toilet regimen is controversial, because the type and duration of

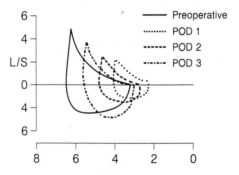

FIGURE 4-3. A patient with mild COPD underwent cholecystectomy through a right subcostal incision. He was coached preoperatively to achieve maximal effort on spirometry, and these data were recorded by plotting inhaled and exhaled flow against volume. Lung volume data also were recorded using a helium dilution technique. Pulmonary function was again measured on the first 3 postoperative days, but only after careful administration of intravenous narcotic to relieve pain. The flow-volume loops were positioned on a single graph to emphasize postoperative changes in lung volume. The first postoperative day, the flow-volume loop is unchanged in shape, but markedly reduced in size. FVC is 50% of peroperative value, even though an attempt to relieve pain and encourage deep breathing preceded the measurement. By the third day, the patient had recovered 80% function.

therapy necessary to modify risk are not standardized. A reasonable approach is listed in Table 4-2. The need for therapy is determined using spirometry,[32] and therapy usually begins the day before surgery.

Postoperative therapeutic maneuvers are designed to reclaim lung volume. The characteristic decrease in FRC results in ventilation-perfusion ($\dot{V}/\dot{Q}$) abnormalities. The lung is at lower resting and lower inflation volumes, but still perfused, which results in low $\dot{V}/\dot{Q}$ and increased intrapulmonary shunting. The resulting hypoxemia may be reversed by deep lung inflation.[34] Bartlett and colleagues[34] used a spirometer to encourage patients to achieve sustained maximal spontaneous inspiration. The device incorporated a mechanism to count the number of times a patient inspired the desired volume, acting as an incentive. When appropriately coached, patients performed the repeated, sustained maximal inspirations necessary to sustain arterial oxygenation and to maintain lung function. Used hourly, this technique improves outcome in most patients.

Upper abdominal surgery is associated with the greatest loss of lung function, suggesting possible harm to the diaphragm due to surgery. Several investigators have reported marked changes in diaphragmatic muscular function after upper abdominal surgery that do not occur after abdominal or nonabdominal procedures.[35,36] The reasons for these changes are unclear, but appear to include local irritation and inflammation. Animal studies reveal that diaphragmatic muscle function can be induced by esophageal or vagal stimulation, suggesting an inhibitory neural reflex. Ford and associates[36] noted a shift in patient breathing patterns: With changes in diaphragm movement, rib-cage breathing increases as abdominal movement decreased. Patients could voluntarily revert to diaphragmatic breathing on command, however, suggesting that an inhibitory neural reflex may suppress diaphragmatic function.

Anesthetic Management

The ability of the anesthesiologist to participate in postoperative pain management of nonthoracic surgical patients may be an important factor in improved outcome. Intercostal nerve blocks improve postoperative pain, but do not improve lung volumes.[37] Epidural opiates appear to produce better pain relief with fewer postoperative pulmonary complications than traditional opiate administration and dosing patterns.[38,39] However, two recent studies report no difference in postoperative pulmonary function or in the incidence of postoperative pulmonary complications with epidural and parenteral opiate analgesia.[40,41] In general, epidural analgesia provides superior pain relief and more normal breathing patterns. The respiratory depressant effects of the opiates require carefully titrated dosing and close monitoring, especially in the elderly.[42]

In conclusion, preoperative assessment of candidates for upper abdominal surgery should be simple, requiring only spirometry and arterial blood-gas analysis. Severe limitations in baseline pulmonary function may indicate the need for postoperative ventilatory support. Moderate impairment indicates increased risk, and preoperative therapy may improve outcome. Postoperative respiratory therapy and pain management strategies can be designed to return pulmonary function to baseline and to decrease the incidence of postoperative pulmonary complications.

References

1. Gaensler EA, Cusell DW, Lindgren I, et al: The role of pulmonary insufficiency in mortality and invalidism following surgery for pulmonary tuberculosis. J Thorac Cardiovasc Surg 29:163, 1955
2. Lockwood P. Lung function test results and the risk of post-thoracotomy complications. Respir 30:529, 1973
3. Olsen GN, Block AJ: Pulmonary function testing in evaluation for pneumonectomy. Hospital Practice 8:137, 1973
4. Boysen PG, Block AJ, Moulder PV: Relationship between preoperative pulmonary function tests and complications after thoracotomy. Surg Gynecol Obstetr 52:813, 1981
5. Mittman C: Assessment of operative risk in thoracic surgery. Am Rev Respir Dis 84:197, 1961
6. Boushy SF, Billig DM, North LB, et al: Clinical course related to preoperative and postoperative pulmonary function in patients with bronchogenic carcinoma. Chest 59:383, 1971
7. Miller JI, Grossman GD, Hatcher CR: Pulmonary function test criteria for operability and pulmonary resection. Surg Gynecol Obstetr 153:893, 1981
8. Boysen PG, Block AJ, Olsen GN, et al: Prospective evaluation for pneumonectomy using the Tc^{99} quantitative perfusion lung scan. Chest 72:422, 1977
9. Markos J, Mullan BP, Hillman DR, et al: Preoperative assessment as a predictor of mortality and morbidity after lung resection. Am Rev Respir Dis 139:902, 1989
10. Olsen GN, Block AJ, Swenson EW, et al: Pulmonary function evaluation of the lung resection candidate: A prospective study. Am Rev Respir Dis 111:379, 1975

11. Gass GD, Olsen GN: Preoperative pulmonary function testing to predict postoperative morbidity and mortality. Chest 89:127, 1986
12. Neuhaus H, Cherniak NS: A bronchospirometric method of estimating the effect of pneumonectomy on the maximum breathing capacity. J Thorac Cardiovasc Surg 55:144, 1968
13. Kristerson S, Lindell S et al: Prediction of pulmonary function loss due to pneumonectomy using [133] Xe-radiospirometry. Chest 62:694, 1972
14. Olsen GN, Block AJ et al: Prediction of postpneumonectomy pulmonary function using quantitative macroaggregate lung scanning. Chest 66:13, 1974
15. Bergan F: A simple method for determination of the relative function of the right and left lung. Acta Chir Scan 253 (suppl):58, 1960
16. Marion JM, Alderson PO et al: Unilateral lung function: Comparison of the lateral position test with radionuclide ventilation-perfusion studies. Chest 69:5, 1976
17. Walkup RE, Vossel LF, Griffin JP, et al: Prediction of postoperative pulmonary function with the lateral position test: A prospective study. Chest 77:24, 1980
18. Jay SJ, Stonehill RB, Kiblani SO, et al: Variability of the lateral position test in normal subjects. Am Rev Respir Dis 121:165-67, 1980
19. Schoonover GA, Olsen GN, Habibian MR, et al: Lateral position test and quantitative lung scan in the preoperative evaluation for lung resection. Chest 86:854, 1984
20. Ali ML, Mountain CF, Ewer MS, et al: Predicting loss of pulmonary function after pulmonary resection for bronchogenic carcinoma. Chest 77:337, 1980
21. Harrison RW, Adams WE, Long ET, et al: The clinical significance of cor pulmonale in the prediction of cardiopulmonary reserve following extensive pulmonary resection. J Thorac Surg 36:352-68, 1958
22. Degraff AC, Taylor HF, Ord JW, et al: Exercise limitation following extensive pulmonary resection. J Clin Invest 44:1514, 1965
23. Uggla LG: Indication for and results of thoracic surgery with regard to respiratory and circulatory function tests. Acta Chir Scand 111:197, 1956
24. Stein M, Koots GM, Simon M, Frank EA: Pulmonary evaluation of surgical patients. JAMA 181: 765-70, 1962
25. Fee JH, Holmes EC, Gerwitz HS, et al: Role of pulmonary vascular resistance measurements in preoperative evaluation of candidates for pulmonary resection. J Thorac Cardiovasc Surg 75:519, 1975
26. Reichel J: Assessment of operative risk of pneumonectomy. Chest 62:570, 1972
27. Colman NC, Schraufrasel DE, Rivington RN, et al: Exercise testing in evaluation of patients for lung resection. Am Rev Respir Dis 125:604, 1982
28. Eugene J, Brown SE, Light RW, et al: Maximum oxygen consumption: A physiology guide to pulmonary resection. Am Rev Respir Dis 125:604, 1982
29. Smith TP, Kinasewitz GT, Tucker WY, et al: Exercise capacity as a predictor of post-thoracotomy morbidity. Am Rev Respir Dis 129:730, 1984
30. Stein M, Cassara EL: Preoperative pulmonary evaluation and therapy for surgery patients. JAMA 211:787, 1970

31. Latimer RG, Dickman M, Day WC, et al: Ventilatory patterns and pulmonary complications after upper abdominal surgery determined by preoperative and postoperative computerized spirometry and blood gas analysis. Am J Surg 122:622, 1971

32. Gracey DR, Divertie MB, Didier EP: Preoperative pulmonary preparation of patients with chronic obstructive pulmonary disease. Chest 61:59, 1979

33. Millegde JS, Nunn JF: Criteria of fitness for anesthesia in patients with chronic obstructive lung disease. Br Med J 3:670, 1975

34. Bartlett RH, Brennan ML, Gazzaniga AB, et al.: Studies on pathogenesis and prediction of postoperative pulmonary complications. Surg Gynecol Obstetr 137:925, 1973

35. Tahir AH, George RB, Weill H, et al: Effects of abdominal surgery upon diaphragmatic function and regional ventilation. Int Surg 58:337, 1973

36. Ford GT, Whitelaw WA, Rosenal TW, et al: Diaphragm function after upper abdominal surgery in humans. Am Rev Respir Dis 127:431, 1983

37. Jakobeon S, Ivarsson J: Effects of intercostal nerve blocks (etidocaine 0.5%) on chest wall mechanics in cholecystectomized patients. Acta Anaesthesiol Scand 21:497, 1977

38. Spence AA, Smith G: Postoperative analgesia and lung function: A comparison of morphine with extradural block. Brit J Anaesth 43:144, 1971

39. Pflug AE, Murphy TM, Butler SH, et al: The effects of postoperative epidural analgesia on pulmonary therapy and pulmonary complications. Anesthesiol 41:8, 1974

40. Jayr C, Mollie A, Bourgain JL, Alarcon J, et al: Postoperative pulmonary complications: General anesthesia with postoperative parenteral morphine compared with epidural analgesia. Surg 104:57, 1987

41. Hjortso NC, Neumann P, Frosig F, et al: A controlled study of the effect of epidural analgesia with local anesthetics and morphine on morbidity after abdominal surgery. Acta Anaesthesiol Scand 29:790, 1985

42. Catley DM, Thornton M, Jordan C, et al: Pronounced, episodic oxygen desaturation in the postoperative period: Its association with ventilatory pattern and analgesic regimen. Anesthesiol 63:20, 1985

43. Candler L: Physiologic assessment and management of the preoperative patient with pulmonary emphysema. Am J Cardiol 12:324, 1963

Robert G. Merin

5 | Preoperative Cardiovascular Medications

In this chapter, I will discuss the significance and importance of cardiovascular medications in assessing the condition of a patient with cardiovascular disease and in preparing the patient for elective anesthesia and surgery. Consequently, I will be discussing only chronic cardiovascular medications and have organized the chapter according to the pharmacology of these medications. For each group of drugs, in addition to the pharmacology, I will comment on the advisability of continuing or discontinuing the use of each drug in the group during the perioperative period. In some cases, I may suggest that a specific drug should be initiated preoperatively in certain patient populations by the anesthesiologist. The categories of drugs I will discuss include drugs acting on or through the sympathetic nervous system; calcium channel-blocking (CCB) drugs; angiotensin-converting enzyme inhibitor (ACEI) drugs; antiarrhythmic drugs; inotropic drugs; vasodilators; diuretics; and, finally, monoamine oxidase inhibitor (MAOI) drugs.

DRUGS ACTING ON OR THROUGH THE SYMPATHETIC NERVOUS SYSTEM

Before discussing agonists and antagonists of the sympathetic nervous system, it is necessary to make a few brief comments about recent advances in adrenergic receptor physiology. In general, sympathetic nervous system activation is designed to prepare the body for emergency situations (fight or flight). Consequently, there is general increase in the function of the cardiovascular and respiratory systems and diversion of blood flow away from less essential organ systems, such as the gastrointestinal and genitourinary systems. Metabolism also is stimulated to provide more fuel for bodily function in the form of glucose and fatty acids. The early categorization of sympathetic nervous receptors noted that alpha receptor activity produced predominantly peripheral vasoconstriction, whereas beta agonism resulted in both cardiac stimulation and relaxation of various smooth muscle beds, including the vascular, the bronchial and even the uterine bed. More recently, both receptor systems have been subdivided. Beta$_1$ receptors primarily mediate the effect of adrenergic agonists on cardiac function, including rate of contraction (chronotropic), rate of conduction of cardiac impulses (dromotropic), and force of contraction of cardiac muscle (inotropic). On the other hand, the beta$_2$ receptors primarily modulate the relaxation of vascular, bronchial, and uterine smooth muscle. Recently, however, it has become apparent that beta$_2$ receptors also may mediate cardiac activity. This observation may assume some therapeutic importance with the demonstration that continued high intensity sympathetic stimulation similar to that in chronic congestive heart failure results in what has been termed "down regulation," that is, decreased density and responsiveness of the receptors.[1] Recently, it has been shown that down regulation in terminal heart failure in humans applies only to beta$_1$ receptors and that the density of beta$_2$ receptors appears to change little in failing human hearts.[2] Consequently, drugs which are predominantly beta$_2$ agonists are more effective in stimulating the inotropic adrenergic response in failing hearts than in normal hearts. The initial division of alpha receptors into alpha$_1$ and alpha$_2$ types delineated an alpha$_2$ receptor in the preganglionic sympathetic nerve terminal which was responsible for a negative feedback mechanism; as sympathetic stimulation occurred, alpha$_2$ agonism by the neurally released norepinephrine served to decrease further norepinephrine release from the nerve terminal. However, it has recently become apparent that alpha$_2$ receptors are more widely distributed. One of the areas where alpha$_2$ agonism is important is in the central nervous system, where stimulation reduces sympathetic outflow and hence acts systemically as a sympathetic inhibitor. Consequently, alpha$_2$ agonists have proved to be rather important antihypertensive drugs and alpha$_2$ antagonists may have the opposite effect; that is, they tend to stimulate the sympathetic nervous system. In addition, there definitely are postsynaptic alpha$_2$ receptors in the peripheral circulation which may be responsible for the alpha agonism from exogenous intravenously used sympathomimetic agents.[3]

Beta-Adrenergic Agonist Drugs

The beta agonist drugs have been used primarily for their chronotropic and inotropic effects on the heart. In most circumstances, the beta$_1$ receptor agonists are thought to be responsible for the therapeutic effect. Since no primary beta$_1$ agonist is effective by the gastrointestinal route because of enzymatic breakdown in the gut, the major chronic use for beta-adrenergic agonists is in the treatment of bronchospasm. The beta$_2$-selective drugs such as metaproterenol and albuterol are widely used for treatment and prophylaxis of bronchial asthma, both in tablet form and through nebulization to the respiratory tract. The influence of these drugs on assessment and preparation of the cardiac patient is outside the scope of this chapter. As mentioned earlier, however, there is some ongoing investigation about the use of beta$_2$ receptor agonists in treating chronic congestive heart failure. At the present time, this work is still investigational. Consequently, it is unlikely that patients who are taking beta$_2$ agonists for their cardiac effect will be presenting for surgery in great numbers.

Beta-Adrenergic Antagonists (Beta Blockers)[4]

During the 1970s, beta blockers were the most widely used cardioactive compounds in the world. In the 1980s, the use of calcium channel blockers caught up with and perhaps surpassed them, but the beta blockers are still widely used. The major difference between the various beta-adrenergic blocking drugs lies primarily in their pharmacokinetics and what have been called their associated side effects. In addition to beta antagonism, these drugs also may produce some membrane-stabilizing activity (local anesthetic activity), intrinsic sympathomimetic activity, or partial agonism (PAA), and may be selective for either the beta$_1$ or the beta$_2$ receptor. Although, the local anesthetic effect was initially thought to be an important determinant of their putative negative inotropic effect, it has become apparent that this effect is only important in very high doses, usually outside the clinical range. There has been considerable controversy about the importance of the properties of partial agonism and receptor selectivity. Currently, two of the available beta blockers, pindolol and acebutolol, produce partial agonism (Table 5-1). This activity has been said to produce less decrease in heart rate and less negative inotropic effect in patients with chronic congestive heart failure. It is also possible that patients with bronchospastic disease and peripheral vascular disease may benefit from some intrinsic beta$_2$ agonism in these drugs. However, the data thus far are relatively inconclusive. Theoretically, beta$_1$ selectivity would also permit the use of such drugs for treatment of bronchospasm and peripheral vascular spasm. The beta$_2$ agonism

TABLE 5-1. Beta-Adrenergic Blocking Drugs

	Potency	B-1 Sel*	PAA*	MSA*	Lip. Sol.	Hep. Metab.	$t^{1/2}B$* (hr)
Propranolol (Inderal)	1	−	−	+	High	High	2–4
Timolol (Blocadren)	6	−	−	−	Moderate	High	4–6
Nadolol (Corgard)	0.8	−	−	−	Low†	Low†	16–24†
Metoprolol (Lopressor)	1	+ +†	−	−	Moderate	High	2.5–4.5
Atenolol (Tenormin)	1	+ +†	−	−	Low†	Low†	6–9†
Pindolol (Visken)	6	−	+ + +†	+	Moderate	Moderate	3–5
Acebutolol (Sectral)	0.3	+†	+†	+	High	High	8–10*
Labetalol Trandate, Normodyne)	0.3	−	−	−	Moderate	High	5–6
Esmolol (Brevibloc)	0.1	+ +†	−	−	Low	Low	0.1†

B-1 sel = beta-1 selective; *PAA* = partial agonist activity; *MSA* = membrane stabilizing activity; $t^{1/2}B$ = elimination half-life
*Active metabolite, diacetol
†Significant difference from propranolol

of the circulating catecholamines and sympathetic stimulation may produce some bronchodilation and vasodilation in such patients. Drugs which block these beta$_2$ effects worsen these disease processes. Unfortunately, all the beta$_1$ selective drugs at present are only selective, and in higher doses also produce beta$_2$ agonism, so that the drugs must be used with great caution in patients with broncho- and vasospasm. In instances where the negative chronotrophic (bradycardic) effect of the drugs may be important, such as protection in patients with ischemic heart disease, beta$_1$ selectivity in these drugs may not be desirable.[5] The two drugs which have been shown to provide some protection against extension of acute myocardial infarctions, propranolol and timolol, are both nonselective blockers. In addition, the epinephrine-produced hypokalemia is probably beta$_2$ receptor-mediated and, if it is important to prevent this effect, a selective beta$_1$ antagonist would not be the drug of choice.[6]

The pharmacokinetics of this class of drugs appears to be related to their lipid solubility. The drugs with moderate or high lipid solubility are metabolized predominantly by the liver and tend to have a relatively short duration of action. By contrast, those agents with low lipid solubility appear to be excreted by the kidneys and tend to be longer acting. Another consequence of hepatic metabolism is a prominent first pass hepatic extraction, resulting in considerably lower and relatively unpredictable plasma levels when these drugs are given orally, than would be expected from an equivalent intravenous dose. Renal function has little effect on the kinetics of the highly lipid-soluble hepatically metabolized beta blockers. On the other hand, the kinetics of the longer acting, less lipid-soluble drugs, such as atenolol and nadolol, are sensitive to renal function.

Drugs

The associated pharmacologic properties of the beta-adrenergic drugs and some kinetic considerations appear in Table 5-1. Most of these drugs are metabolized predominantly by the liver and thus have a high first pass extraction and a relatively short elimination half life (propranolol, timolol, metoprolol, pindolol, acebutolol, labetalol). Nadolol and atenolol are both excreted primarily by the kidney and have a long elimination half life; the newest beta-blocker, esmolol, is unique in that it is hydrolyzed by plasma esterases and therefore is ultra short-acting. It is useful primarily in the acute management of patients and will not be considered further in this chapter. As mentioned earlier, the membrane-stabilizing activity of these drugs is unimportant. Three of the drugs, metoprolol, atenolol, and acebutolol, have beta$_1$ selectivity, although acebutolol is less selective. Two drugs, pindolol and acebutolol, possess partial agonist activity. Again, acebutolol is less potent. Labetalol is unique in that it possesses some alpha-adrenergic blocking activity. It is generally thought that this activity is approximately one tenth that of its beta-blocking activity, so that labetalol should be considered primarily a beta blocker.

Drug Uses

One recent review reported 51 different clinical syndromes for which beta-adrenergic blockade is reported to be useful![7] However, the most popular use for these drugs is for cardiovascular diseases. Certainly, the two most common cardiovascular diseases, ischemic heart disease (coronary artery disease) and essential hypertension, are the most common diseases to be treated with beta blockers. Calcium-blocking drugs have become more popular, especially for patients with ischemic heart disease and angina pectoris, and many patients are being treated with both drugs. Another syndrome for which beta-blocking drugs have been effective is hypertrophic cardiomyopathy, both of the left (asymmetric septal hypertrophy) and the right ventricle (pulmonary infundibular stenosis and tetralogy of Fallot). Of course, supraventricular tachycardias, slowing of ventricular response, atrial fibrillation, and flutter are other areas where beta blockers may be indicated. The myriad of other syndromes includes thyrotoxicosis, glaucoma, central nervous system initiated muscular tremors, and drug abuse.

Preoperative Considerations

Although an early report suggested that a beta blocker should be discontinued before elective surgery, I believe there can be no doubt today that patients who are taking beta blockers chronically should be continued on the beta blockers, not only up until surgery, but probably throughout the perioperative period.[8] Certainly, in the patient with ischemic heart disease, the most effective treatment for tachyarrhythmias is still beta blockade, and tachyarrhythmias are especially deleterious to myocardial oxygen balance. One study has even shown that beginning beta block therapy in previously untreated patients may be advantageous during the perioperative period.[9] In any event, the current state of the art is that patients who are receiving beta blockers must continue to receive them, at least on the day of surgery and perhaps through the first few postoperative days.

Beta blockers do generally decrease liver blood flow and thus the elimination half-life of any drug metabolized by the liver may be prolonged when given in combination with beta blockers. The other major problem with drug interaction involves other cardioactive drugs. In particular, the combination of the beta blockers and calcium blockers must be viewed with caution. This should not be surprising since these drugs have some similar actions and often are prescribed for the same diseases. In particular, the combination may undesirably prolong atrial ventricular conduction, resulting in complete heart block. The drugs appear to be better tolerated when given together orally than when given intravenously. The same precautions, particularly for atrioventricular block, are true for most of the Class I antiarrhythmic drugs and digitalis. On the other hand, beta blockers have proved 'to be efficacious for treating digitalis toxicity.

Alpha-Adrenergic Agonists

A major use of alpha-adrenergic agonists, of course, is in the acute management of hypotension, especially secondary to sympathetic blockade (regional anesthesia). The anesthesiologist is usually seeking alpha$_1$ agonism in such cases. However, for chronic therapy alpha$_2$ agonists have become popular in recent years, for treatment not of hypotension, but, rather, of hypertension (as mentioned earlier, central alpha$_2$ agonism results in a decrease in sympathetic outflow and thus produces a sympatholytic effect). The original antihypertensive drug acting through this mechanism, although initially this was not realized, was alpha methyldopa (Aldomet). The major metabolite of this compound, alpha methyl norepinephrine, is a potent alpha$_2$ agonist, and this is certainly the mechanism of action of this drug. More recently, other alpha$_2$ agonist drugs have been approved for use in the hypertensive patient, including clonidine (Catapres), guanabenz (Wytensin), and guanfacine (Tenex). The clinical pharmacology of these drugs is practically identical. As with most other drugs which interfere in sympathetic nervous function, the primary problem is hypotension, particularly in patients who are hypovolemic or vasodilated (regional or general anesthetics). Careful attention to fluid volume status and therapy is necessary during the perioperative period.

Preoperative Considerations

Soon after the release of clonidine, the problem of rebound hypertension in the postoperative period was identified.[10] This was particularly troublesome to clinicians because no parenteral dose form of clonidine was available. However, the problem appears not to occur if clonidine is continued up to and on the day of surgery. In addition, since alpha methyldopa has the same mechanism of action, this drug can be used parenterally to cover patients who are being treated with clonidine. Although previously demonstrated for alpha methyldopa, the particular ability of $alpha_2$ agonist drugs both to decrease anesthetic requirements and to smooth the cardiovascular lability frequently seen during anesthesia in hypertensive patients has recently been studied.[11] Several groups have demonstrated that treating patients with a single dose of oral clonidine 1–2 hours before the initiation of anesthesia has resulted in a more favorable anesthetic course.[12–15] With the advent of even more selective and potent $alpha_2$ agonist drugs, it may become common practice to medicate hypertensive patients with these drugs preoperatively to produce a more stable perioperative course.

Alpha-Adrenergic Antagonists

Alpha-adrenergic antagonists will be effective antihypertensive drugs only in cases having significant sympathetic nervous system activity. However, if these drugs are given alone under these circumstances, there will be appreciable tachycardia because the beta effects of sympathetic activity will be unopposed. Although there is considerable controversy about the specific role of the sympathetic nervous system in essential hypertension, $alpha_1$-adrenergic receptor-blocking drugs have been introduced for the treatment of hypertension. The first of these is prazosin (Minipress). The selective $alpha_1$-blocking activity means that the $alpha_2$ negative feedback on the prejunctional sympathetic nerve terminal is still intact and tachycardia is less often a problem. Another piperazine derivative, terazosin (Hytrin), also is available. There also is an indole derivative, indoramin. The latter also is an $alpha_1$ antagonist but possesses some Class III and, in higher doses, Class I antiarrhythmic properties. However, these do not appear to be important in clinical practice.

Catecholamine-Depleting Drugs

This category of drugs actually introduced effective antihypertensive therapy decades ago with the use of the rauwolfia alkaloids. However, because of their wide spectrum of side effects in addition to hypotension (they also were the first effective major tranquilizers), these drugs have essentially been replaced by more specific catecholamine-depleting drugs, particularly the guanethidine drugs. The latter do not deplete central nervous system (CNS) catecholamine stores as the rauwolfia alkaloids do, and affect only the peripheral nervous system. Consequently, CNS side effects are unusual. The drugs include the original guanethidine (Ismelin) and the most recently approved, guanadrel (Hylorel). Although its pharmacology is similar to that of the guanethidine drugs, guanadrel is better absorbed by oral administration, faster in onset, and shorter in duration.[16]

ANGIOTENSIN-CONVERTING ENZYME INHIBITORS (ACEI)

The renin-angiotensin system aids in maintaining body blood pressure and water homeostasis. The major end product of the system, angiotensin II, is a potent vasoconstrictor and stimulates the release of aldosterone from the adrenal cortex. Aldosterone causes salt and water retention by the kidney. Angiotensin is produced by the following mechanism: the juxtaglomerular cells of the renal cortex secrete a proteolytic enzyme called renin, which cleaves a protein produced in the liver to a decapeptide angiotensin I that is a mild vasoconstrictor. Angiotensin I is converted almost immediately to angiotensin II by the activity of the angiotensin-converting enzyme (ACE) which is located predominantly in the endothelial tissue of the lung. Angiotensin II, in addition to being a vasoconstrictor, facilitates the prejunctional release of norepinephrine at the sympathetic nerve terminal. It also directly decreases tubular reabsorption of sodium, increases ADH and ACTH secretion, and stimulates the secretion of aldosterone. A minority of patients with hypertensive vascular disease may have high circulating plasma renin levels, and administration of ACEI drugs which interfere with the formation of activity of angiotensin II will decrease blood pressure. Three such drugs are presently available: the first of these is captopril (Capoten) and the newer ACEI drugs are enalapril (Vasotec) and lisinopril (Prinivil). Enalapril is effective primarily because it is hydrolyzed to the ethyl ester or enalaprilate. This metabolite is now available in the intravenous form and is known as Vasotec IV. Because the effect of enalapril is dependent on metabolism, its pharmacokinetics are relatively unpredictable. Generally, its onset of action is considerably slower than that of captopril. Lisinopril is not a pro-drug, but is relatively slow in onset, like enalapril. The slow onset of the two newer drugs may decrease the first-dose hypotension that has been reported with captopril. Interestingly, though, these drugs are effective not only in treating high renin hypertension but also in normal and low renin states. In addition, they have been very effective in treating congestive heart failure when vasodilation is desired and, in particular, appear to produce less tolerance than other vasodilators, and fewer renal effects.[17]

Preoperative Considerations

With the sympatholytic drugs, the major problem is peripheral vasodilation, which is accentuated in the presence of other vasodilators (anesthetics) or hypovolemia.

To my knowledge, there are no specific preoperative problems in patients on ACEI drugs. As with all sympatholytic or vasodilator drugs, patients may be more sensitive to hypovolemia. The availability of the enalaprilate intravenous formulation means that ACEI treatment can now be maintained through the perioperative period in patients who are unable to take oral medications.

CALCIUM CHANNEL-BLOCKING (CCB) DRUGS

Given the ubiquitous nature of the calcium ion as a second or third messenger in mediating cell activity, it is not surprising that drugs which interfere in calcium homeostasis may be useful in a variety of disease states, particularly those involving excess cardiovascular activity.

Pharmacology[18]

Although these drugs have been referred to as "calcium antagonists," they are not actually pharmacologic antagonists of the calcium ion. Rather, they interfere with the passage of calcium ions through the cell membrane (there may be some effect on calcium channels on interior cellular membranes as well, but this is still controversial). Since the influx of calcium ion from the high concentration in the extracellular fluid through the cell membrane to raise the normally low concentration intracellularly (less than 10-6 M) is the major event that initiates contraction of all muscle, it is logical that the major use of calcium channel-blocking drugs involves interference with the contraction of various types of muscle. It is also in keeping with the physiology that effects of channel blockers on skeletal muscle are minimal, because skeletal muscle does not depend as much as cardiac and smooth muscle on calcium ion influx through the cell membrane to initiate muscle contraction. Consequently, CCBs primarily affect cardiac and smooth muscle contraction. Because the calcium ion provides the major current for the automatic and conducting tissues of the heart (S-A and A-V nodes), these drugs also have an effective antiarrhythmic action. Since their primary effect is not on the electrical activity of actual heart muscle, or the Purkinje fibers, the major use of these drugs is in treating supraventricular arrhythmias, particularly paroxysmal supraventricular arrhythmias.

TABLE 5-2. Calcium Channel-blocking Drugs: Clinical Effects

	Anti-arrhythmic	Cardiac Depression	Tachy-cardia	Vasodilation		
				Syst.	Coronary	Cerebral
Verapamil (Isoptin, Calan)	+ + +	+ +	−	+	+	+
Diltiazem (Cardizem)	+ +	+	−	+ +	+ +	+ +
Nifedipine (Procardia)	−	+	+ +	+ + +	+ + +	+ + +
Nicardipine (Cardene)	−	−	+ +	+ + +	+ + +	+ + +
Nimodipine	−	−	+ +	+ +	+ +	+ + +

Unlike the beta-adrenergic blocking drugs which have a near-rigid structure activity relationship, several different chemical formulations have potent calcium channel-blocking activities. The original papaverine derivatives, verapamil and D-600, were the prototype CCB drugs. However, most of the newer drugs are dihydroperidines of the nifedipine type. The diphenyl alkylamines such as diltiazem also belong to this class of drugs. Verapamil and nifedipine are at opposite ends of the spectrum (Table 5-2). Nifedipine is primarily a vasodilator drug with minimal effects on cardiac muscle and electrophysiology in intact animals and humans. Verapamil, on the other hand, has vasodilatory properties, but also is a potent antiarrhythmic and direct depressant of cardiac muscle. Diltiazem appears to have effects intermediate to those of nifedipine and verapamil, possessing all the CCB properties of both, but producing more prominent vasodilation than nifedipine.

Drug Uses

The clinical uses for these drugs are remarkably similar to those of the beta blockers. As with the beta blockers, the first FDA-approved indication was for the treatment of arrhythmias, in this case, supraventricular arrhythmias. Verapamil and, to a lesser extent, diltiazem are currently the drugs of choice for conversion of paroxysmal supraventricular arrhythmias. As with the beta blockers, the second FDA-approved indication was for the treatment of ischemic heart disease (IHD). The major advantage of these drugs over the beta blockers for the treatment of IHD is that they are coronary vasodilators. Thus, in addition to decreasing myocardial oxygen demand by decreasing blood pressure, heart rate, and force of myocardial contraction, they also may improve supply through coronary vasodilation if coronary vasospasm is a part of the disease. The third FDA-approved use, as with the beta blockers, is for the treatment of hypertension. Like most antihypertensive drugs, the calcium blockers are not miracle drugs. By trial and error, patients who appear to be particularly responsive to CCBs rather than other antihypertensive drugs can be identified. Again, like the beta blockers, if patients with hypertension also have ischemic heart disease, then the CCBs may be a particularly valuable therapy. The CCBs also are being used often in concert with the beta blockers to treat hypertrophic cardiomyopathies, although this use is not FDA-approved. Because they are smooth muscle relaxants, they also are under investigation for treatment of various smooth muscle spasm conditions such as bronchospasm, vasospasm, and premature labor. Their efficacy in treating these conditions has not been well established. However, it is important to note that even if these drugs are not therapeutic for the smooth muscle spastic disease or premature labor, the CCBs can be used safely for other indications in patients with both bronchospasm and vasospasm, unlike the beta blockers, which are relatively contraindicated in these diseases.

Drugs

There are basically three types of CCBs. Verapamil and diltiazem are the only currently approved drugs in their chemical category and, as indicated earlier, they are similar in activity, diltiazem being a somewhat better vasodilator. The dihydroperidine drugs with nifedipine as the parent now have yielded two new FDA-approved compounds; both nicardipine (Cardene) and nimodipine have been released for use. Nicardipine is very similar to nifedipine. For the anesthesiologist, it was hoped that because nicardipine is not light-sensitive, as nifedipine is, it would be released for intravenous use. However, it was initially released for oral use only. Some of the experimental investigations suggested that nicardipine might be a better coronary vasodilator, having fewer cardiac depressant properties than nifedipine, but nifedipine has minimal cardiac depressant properties anyway. The drug has been released for the treatment of both hypertension and ischemic heart disease. Nimodipine, on the other hand, appears to be a more specific cerebral vasodilator than some of the other dihydroperidines. It has been released specifically for cerebral protection in patients with cerebral vascular disease.[19]

Preoperative Considerations

As with any drug which produces cardiovascular depression, there has been some controversy about the advisability of continuing calcium channel-blocking drugs throughout the perioperative period.[20] Although rebound effects from withdrawal of the CCBs have not been as prominent as those seen with the BABs, the experimental evidence on the interaction between the calcium channel-blocking drugs and surgery and anesthesia nevertheless suggests that if the drugs are having a favorable effect in the patient, they should be continued through the perioperative period. In highly-instrumented open chest animals, verapamil (in particular) and diltiazem can produce major cardiovascular depression in concert with potent inhalation anesthetics. However, in less invasive closed chest preparations, clinical doses of both CCBs and anesthetics have produced minimal cardiovascular depression. Only with high doses of both classes of drugs have major cardiovascular effects been seen. In particular, the combination of verapamil and enflurane seems to produce a higher incidence of atrioventricular conduction disturbances than other drug combinations. Chronic administration of these drugs appears to produce even less cardiovascular depression, even with relatively high plasma levels of verapamil in one experimental preparation.[21]

Considering the increased importance of preventing and treating perioperative myocardial ischemia and the demonstration that much of this ischemia is not related to altered hemodynamics, it would seem that the calcium blocking drugs might be desirable for myocardial protection during surgery and anesthesia in patients with ischemic heart disease because of their prominent coronary vasodilating activity. Two studies, however, have suggested that patients with ischemic heart disease treated only with calcium channel blockers have a higher incidence of perioperative ischemia than comparable patients treated with beta blockers or the combination of beta blockers and calcium blockers.[22,23] However, the actual degree of calcium block and compliance was not assessed in these studies. Whether or not intravenous administration of calcium blockers in the perioperative period or specific immediate preoperative oral administration might be protective has not been determined.

ANTI-ARRHYTHMIC DRUGS

Most cardiologists and electrophysiologists classify antiarrhythmic drugs using the original classification of Singh and Vaughn-Williams. However, the introduction of new drugs, particularly in Class I (Table 5-3), has made the classification less rigid.[24] In general, Class I drugs are primarily sodium channel-blocking compounds which have been subdivided into 1-A, the quinidine-like drugs, and 1-B, the lidocaine-like drugs. Singh now also suggests a 1-C category in which he includes some of the newer 1-A drugs, such as encainide and flecainide. In general, the 1-A drugs tend to produce more widespread depression of cardiac conductive activities, including the atrioventricular node and the His–Purkinje system. In addition, they produce more direct cardiac depression at the lower plasma levels than the 1-

TABLE 5-3.   Anti-arrhythmic Drugs

I. Sodium channel blocking drugs

    A. Quinidine, procainamide (Norpace)
       Prolong repolarization, rate-dependent
    B. Lidocaine, mexiletine (Mexitil), tocainide (Tonocard)
       Voltage-dependent
    C. Encainide (Enkaid), flecainide (Tambocor)

II. Beta-adrenergic blocking drugs

    (see Table 5-1)

III. Bretylium tosylate (Bretylol), amiodarone (Cardarone)

    Prolong action-potential duration

IV. Calcium channel blocking drugs

    (see Table 5-2)

B drugs. The major difference between the new 1-B drugs, mexilitine and tocainide, and their parent compound, lidocaine, is resistance to both gut enzymes and liver biotransformation, meaning that the latter two drugs can be given orally, unlike lidocaine. Class II and Class IV drugs, of course, have already been discussed. The Class III drugs are particularly vexing, inasmuch as the mechanism of action is still unclear. The major drug in this category that the clinician is apt to encounter is amiodarone (Cordarone). This drug is usually the last-ditch attempt at treating complex ventricular arrhythmias, particularly paroxysmal ventricular tachycardia and fibrillation. Most patients who are treated with amiodarone will eventually require surgical ablation of their arrhythmias and present specialized problems which are beyond the scope of this discussion. Of particular import in the pharmacology of amiodarone is the fact that, for full clinical effect, the drug needs to be given for at least two weeks and, probably, a month to build up tissue levels. Once these levels are obtained, it is not clear how long it takes for the drug effects to dissipate after the drug is discontinued. There are some indications that it may never be completely eliminated from the body. Consequently, a patient taking amiodarone must be considered to have the drug's effects almost permanently. A discussion of the indications for the various antiarrhythmic drugs is beyond the scope of this presentation. The anesthesiologist should have some idea of the comparative pharmacology of the various antiarrhythmics (see Table 5-3).

Preoperative Considerations[25]

As with all cardioactive drugs, if the drug is having a beneficial effect, it should be continued throughout the patient's perioperative course. The quinidine-like drugs are likely to interact with potent inhalation anesthetics to produce greater cardiovascular deficit, particularly cardiac depression. In addition, since the inhalation anesthetics also produce some interference in liver biotransformation of drugs, and since most of these drugs are biotransformed in the liver, the dose of the drug should be decreased during the perioperative period. Of particular import may be amiodarone. There has been at least one report of major cardiovascular depression occurring postoperatively in a patient given amiodarone therapy.[26] Great caution should be taken in anesthetizing patients who are taking amiodarone.

POSITIVE INOTROPIC DRUGS

Digitalis

As one of the world's experts has recently said, "Although few clinicians would challenge the efficacy of cardiac glycosides in patients with congestive heart failure complicated by supraventricular tachyarrhythmias such as atrial fibrillation, the efficacy of digitalis in the management of heart failure in the presence of normal sinus rhythm has been called into question."[27] Many cardiologists today believe digitalis is an obsolete drug and, consequently, fewer patients are coming to surgery and anesthesia treated with digitalis glycosides. There are two major reasons for this. In the first place, there is some evidence to suggest that in the absence of supraventricular tachyarrhythmias, the effect of digitalis on the pumping ability of the heart is related primarily to extra-cardiac effects (vagal and sympatholytic), and that such therapy is more logically produced by treating patients with vasodilators or drugs which specifically decrease heart rate. The second reason is that digitalis definitely has recognized toxicity that often is difficult to predict and recognize. Anorexia, nausea, and vomiting probably are related to central stimulation of chemoreceptors. The sometimes troublesome vasoconstriction may be related to central sympathetic stimulation. However, the most serious toxic effect of digitalis is certainly arrhythmias, which usually are ventricular in origin and may be very troublesome. The availability of serum digoxin levels has helped in recognition and treatment of digitalis toxicity, but cannot be accepted as the sole arbiter of the presence or action of toxicity.[27] In addition to the availability of serum digoxin levels, there is now a very effective treatment obtained through digoxin's specific FAB fragments, which bind the digoxin and result in spectacular relief of digitalis toxicity. On the other hand, there continue to be impressive studies documenting the effectiveness of digitalis in chronic congestive heart failure. A recently reported large scale multi-institutional double-blind study demonstrated that digoxin alone was equal or superior to milrinone or a combination of digoxin and milrinone in treating congestive heart failure.[28] The same expert on digitalis suggested, "A consensus now exists that patients with dilated failing hearts and impaired systolic function often manifesting an S_3 gallop have subjective and objective improvement after receiving digitalis, whereas patients with elevated filling pressures due to reduced ventricular compliance but with preserved systolic function at rest are usually not appropriate candidates for digitalis therapy unless supraventricular tachycardia is a concomitant problem."[27] Although many patients with chronic congestive heart failure can benefit from treatment with vasodilators, including ACEI drugs, alpha blocking drugs, and direct vasodilators, digoxin nevertheless remains an important positive inotropic drug for chronic treatment of the patient with impaired systolic function. Of course, the patient with the combination of chronic congestive failure and supraventricular arrhythmias is a prime candidate for digitalis, inasmuch as the other drugs which are effective in treating supraventricular arrhythmias (calcium blockers, beta blockers, and antiarrhythmics) also tend to decrease ventricular function. The old practice of increasing digitalis dose until toxicity appeared and then backing off can no longer be accepted. Plasma digoxin levels should never exceed 1.5–2.0 ng/ml^{-1}, and monitoring of function, either invasively (PA catheter) or noninvasively (echo and ultrasound), has made therapy at lower doses more efficacious. cious.

Newer Positive Inotropic Drugs[29]

Although there is intense activity in the development of positive inotropic drugs which can be given orally on a chronic basis, to date, none has been approved by the FDA. The bipyridine derivatives, amrinone and milrinone, were the result of such an attempt. These drugs are predominantly phosphodiesterase inhibitors and, consequently, increase intracellular concentration of cyclic AMP as a mechanism of their positive inotropic action. Although they were originally touted as specific for cardiac phosphodiesterase, a major portion of their effectiveness stems from their vasodilating activity and thus, obviously, they also inhibit phosphodiesterase in vascular smooth muscle.[30] However, amrinone has proved to be too toxic on a chronic basis and is only available as an intravenous compound; milrinone, likewise, has not been released for chronic oral use. Consequently, at the present time, patients coming for elective surgery will not be treated with oral bipyridine derivatives unless they are in an investigative protocol. The major advantage of the bipyridines over digitalis is the lack of any effect on cardiac rhythm, so that arrhythmias are never a problem. There is also some indication that these drugs will improve diastolic ventricular function (increase ventricular compliance) in contrast to the digitalis glycosides.

Preoperative Considerations

The early experience in preparing patients for cardiopulmonary bypass suggested that it was important that digitalis be discontinued several days before bypass because of the possibility that significant hypokalemia produced by the bypass might produce ventricular arrhythmias in the digitalized patient. In addition, most of the early bypass patients were having reparative surgery, so that their ventricular function was improved after the operation. Subsequently, we have learned that, in fact, there is probably little depletion of potassium by properly conducted cardiopulmonary bypass and that patients, particularly those whose ventricular function is marginal even for cardiopulmonary bypass, should be maintained on their digitalis. Certainly, patients with chronic congestive failure who are digitalized and coming for elective non-cardiac surgery should be maintained on their digitalis compound. A serum digoxin level should be obtained in the 24 hours before surgery and, if there is evidence of underdigitalization, the surgery should be postponed until the patient is properly digitalized. Of course, if there is evidence of digitalis toxicity, surgery should be postponed until this has been corrected. Although the suggestion was made several decades ago that certain patients might benefit from prophylactic digitalization (particularly elderly patients having pneumonectomies),[31] there has been remarkable resistance to this suggestion. In fact, several studies have demonstrated that preoperative prophylactic digitalization of patients with coronary artery disease resulted in improved function and outcome (decreased incidence of postoperative arrhythmias) in patients not in overt congestive heart failure.[32,33] My opinion is that no patient who is properly digitalized should be withdrawn from digitalis preoperatively and that there may be some indications for preoperative prophylactic digitalization.

DIRECT VASODILATORS

Although one of the first widely used antihypertensive drugs, hydralazine, was, in fact, a direct peripheral vasodilator, these drugs have not achieved widespread use in the treatment of hypertension, principally because of the reflex effects of the vasodilation. All of the direct-acting potent vasodilators have two major side effects, which are generally undesirable.[25] The vasodilation results in tachycardia and fluid retention. Consequently, these drugs often are used in combination with both a beta blocker to treat the tachycardia and a diuretic to combat the fluid retention. Hydralazine (Apresoline) and minoxidil (Minipress) are the two most commonly used, chronically administered, direct-acting vasodilators. For the reasons just noted, the drugs are not widely used. In addition to tachycardia and urinary retention, minoxidil also produces hirsutism and, in fact, is now being marketed for that purpose.

The other widely used direct vasodilators are, of course, the inorganic nitrates. In anesthesiology, we commonly use these drugs for acute reduction in blood pressure and treatment of myocardial ischemia. (As mentioned in the introduction, these uses will not be covered in this presentation.) The nitrates that are used chronically are useful mainly for treatment of ischemic heart disease, not hypertension.[34] Nitroglycerin has been used in various formulations for producing decreased myocardial oxygen demand and coronary vasodilation. Both as a paste and patches applied to the skin, the drug has been very popular. However, absorption of nitroglycerin administered in both forms is uncertain. Other nitrates are commonly administered orally for prolonged treatment or prophylaxis of angina pectoris. There is essentially no difference in the various formulations: isosorbide dinitrate (Isordil), pentaerythritol tetranitrate (Peritrate), erythrityl tetranitrate (Cardilate). All produce an effect in 15–20 minutes that lasts anywhere from 2 to 6 hours. There has been considerable controversy about the efficacy of these drugs. As many studies deny their efficacy as support their use, both for increasing angina threshold and treating the pain of angina pectoris. In addition, there is undeniable evidence that tolerance to the use of oral nitrate compounds develops. Consequently, the chronic continued use of the long-acting nitrates makes little sense. These drugs, if they are to be used, should be used on an intermittent basis, such as every other day, or every third day, or as necessary, rather than as continuous chronic medications.

Preoperative Considerations

The potent vasodilators (hydralazine and minoxidil) can produce a state similar to the drugs that sympathectomize patients. These patients may be more sensitive to other vasodilators and hypovolemia. In addition, if they are used alone, urinary retention may be a problem. A major consideration for use of the nitrates is that a patient who has been taking long-acting nitrates for any period of time may not respond perioperatively to intravenous nitrates, particularly nitroglycerin, for the treatment of myocardial ischemia.

DIURETICS

The major categories of diuretics include osmotic agents, carbonic anhydrase inhibitors, mercurial diuretics, thiazides (and other cortical effect diuretics), potassium-sparing diuretics, and loop diuretics.[35] Osmotic diuretics are used primarily on an acute basis for increasing urine flow or decreasing cellular water content. Carbonic anhydrase inhibitors are useful primarily for very specific circumstances, on an acute basis, and mercurial diuretics have practically disappeared from practice. Consequently, the major classes of diuretics that are administered chronically today are the thiazide, loop, and potassium-sparing diuretics. The potassium-sparing diuretics include spironolactone (Aldactone), triamterene (Dyrenium), and amiloride (Moduretic, Midamor). These drugs are rarely used alone, except for spironolactone, which is used in patients with aldosterone-secreting tumors because spironolactone is a specific aldosterone antagonist. Triamterene is used mostly in combination with thiazide diuretics (Dyazide, Maxide) to decrease the hypokalemia that these diuretics produce. In the past, one of the first line therapies for mild essential hypertension has been the thiazide diuretics. These drugs, although primarily diuretics, also have some vasodilating properties and patients with mild hypertension often can be effectively treated with only small doses of the thiazides. As mentioned earlier, prolonged thiazide administration, in addition to producing the desired sodium and water diuresis, also may result in unwanted loss of potassium ion. Moreover, hyperuricemia and bone marrow depression sometimes can develop. There is a plethora of thiazide type diuretics, with no appreciable advantage over the original thiazides reported for any one of them (Table 5-4).

The most potent diuretics available today are the loop diuretics. The two original compounds, furosemide (Lasix) and ethycrinic acid (Edecrine), have now been joined by bumetanide (Bumex). The latter drug is more potent and might have greater bioavailability, but otherwise produces the same sort of effects. These drugs can produce profound fluid loss and patients can become quite dehydrated. As with the thiazide diuretics, potassium loss is a major consequence. Again, diuretics today often are administered in combination with other antihypertensive drugs or vasodilators and digitalis in patients with congestive heart failure.

Preoperative Considerations

The major problems to be identified in patients taking these drugs are, of course, hypovolemia and hypokalemia. There is a controversy about the significance of chronic hypokalemia for preoperative assessment of patients. There still are no definitive studies on the subject, but several less than ideal surveys suggest that chronic hypokalemia, unless the patient is digitalized, is not a major problem. However, this is one group of drugs in which discontinuance in the preoperative period certainly is harmful to the patient and may be justified.

TABLE 5-4.   Thiazide (Cortical) Diuretics

Trade Name	Generic
Thiazides	
Diuril, Esidrix, Oretic	hydrochlorothiazide
Aquatensen, Enduron	methyclothiazide
Diucardin, Saluron	hydroflumethiazide
Exna	benzthiazide
Metahydrin, Naqua	trichlormethiazide
Renese	polythiazide
Others	
Lozol	indapamide
Zaroxolyn	metolazone

MONOAMINE OXIDASE INHIBITING (MAOI) DRUGS

Although these drugs were originally introduced as antihypertensive agents, they are most commonly prescribed today as antidepressants. Although the introduction of the tricyclic compounds in the 1970s markedly reduced the use of the MAOI drugs, they appear to be making a comeback, because they are more effective than the tricyclics in many severely depressed patients. The old anesthesia literature (largely anecdotal) suggested that these drugs definitely had to be discontinued at least two weeks before elective surgery. The actions of narcotics, barbiturates, and inhalation agents were said to be prolonged and intensified. Circulatory instability was common. A syndrome characterized by excitation, rigidity, hyperpyrexia, shock and coma was reported following the use of narcotics. However, a recent clinical study[36] and two published reviews[37,38] suggest that, as long as certain drugs are avoided, and careful attention is given to patient monitoring, elective surgery may be safely performed in patients continued on MAOI drugs. It must be realized that patients on these drugs often have severe depressive illnesses and run a major risk of suicide. Consequently, discontinuance of the drugs may be life-threatening. Suggestions from the recent reviewers include: examination of liver function because of the possibility of drug-induced abnormalities; generous premedication, particularly with benzodiazepines; beat-to-beat heart rate and blood pressure monitoring; anesthetic techniques which tend to avoid sympathetic stimulation; and avoidance of meperidine, because there is reasonable documentation of deleterious drug interactions. Of course, indirect-acting sympathomimetic amines, such as ephedrine, methamphetamine, and mephentermine, should not be used, because these drugs markedly increase the intraneuronal storage of norepinephrine. Direct-acting sympathomimetic drugs should be titrated very carefully. Finally, again because of the build-up of endogenous norepinephrine, cocaine should probably be avoided.

Preoperative Considerations

I believe that there is no reason to discontinue MAOI drugs in the preoperative period for elective surgery. In fact, there is a rationale based on knowledge of the pharmacology involved that they should be continued through the stressful perioperative period.

SUMMARY

I believe that, with the possible exception of diuretics, any cardioactive medication that benefits the cardiovascular system of a patient should *not* be discontinued during the perioperative period. Patients who are being treated with these potent drugs have serious cardiovascular disease. Consequently, the anesthesiologist managing such patients should take advantage of the therapy that has benefitted them. In addition to understanding the pathophysiology of the disease of our patients, we must be familiar with the pharmacology of the drugs our patients are taking. If the pathophysiology and the pharmacology are understood, then maintaining the patient's optimal therapy through anesthesia and surgery and the recovery period must be in the best interests of the patient and should be the course of action.

References

1. Hedberg A, Kemp FF, Josephson ME, et al: Co-existence of beta$_1$ and beta$_2$-adrenergic receptors in the human heart: Effects of treatment with receptor antagonists or calcium entry blockers. J Pharmacol 234:561, 1985
2. Bristow MR, Ginsburg R, Umans V, et al: Beta$_1$ and beta$_2$-adrenergic receptor subpopulations in non-failing and failing human ventricular myocardium: Coupling of both receptor subtypes to muscle contraction and selective beta$_1$ receptor down-regulation in heart failure. Circ Res 59:297, 1986
3. Merin RG: Pharmacology of the autonomic nervous system. In Miller RD (ed): Anesthesia, 3rd ed. Churchhill Livingstone, 1989 (in press)
4. Merin RG: New drugs: Beta-adrenergic blockers. Seminars in Anesthesia 7:75, 1988
5. Kjekshus JK: Importance of heart rate in determining beta-blocker efficacy in acute and long-term acute myocardial infarction intervention trials. Am J Cardiol 57:43F, 1986
6. Reid JL, Whyte KF, Struthers AD: Epinephrine-induced hypokalemia: The role of beta-adrenoreceptors. Am J Cardiol 57:23F, 1986
7. Frishman WH, Teicher M: Beta-adrenergic blockade: An update. Cardiology 72:280, 1985
8. Rangno RE: Propranolol withdrawal: Practical considerations. Arch Int Med 141:161, 1981
9. Stone JG, Foex P, Sear JW, et al: Myocardial ischemia in undertreated hypertensive patients: Effect of a single small oral dose of a beta-adrenergic blocking agent. Anesthesiology 68:495, 1988

10. Bloor BC, Flacke JW, Flacke WE: Perioperative clonidine withdrawal syndrome. In Reves JG (ed): Common Problems in Cardiac Anesthesia, p 397. Chicago, Yearbook Medical Publishers, 1987

11. Longnecker DE: Alpine anesthesia: Can pretreatment with clonidine decrease the peaks and valleys? Anesthesiology 67:1, 1987

12. Ghignone M, Calvillo O, Quintin L: Anesthesia and hypertension: The effect of clonidine on perioperative hemodynamics in isoflurane requirements. Anesthesiology 67:3, 1987

13. Flacke JW, Bloor BC, Flacke WE, et al: Reduced narcotic requirement by clonidine with improved hemodynamic and adrenergic stability in patients undergoing coronary bypass surgery. Anesthesiology 67:11, 1987

14. Ghignone M, Noe C, Calvillo O, et al: Anesthesia for ophthalmic surgery in the elderly: The effects of clonidine on intraocular pressure, perioperative hemodynamics and anesthetic requirements. Anesthesiology 68:707, 1988

15. Woodcock TE, Millard RK, Dixon J, et al: Clonidine premedication for isoflurane-induced hypotension. Br J Anaesth 60:388, 1988

16. Finnerty FA, Brogben RN: Guanadrel: A review of its pharmacodynamic and pharmacokinetic properties in therapeutic use in hypertension. Drugs 30:21, 1985

17. Packer M: Converting enzyme-inhibition in the management of severe chronic congestive heart failure: Physiologic concepts. J Cardiovasc Pharmaco 10(suppl 7):S9-S16, 1987

18. Kapur PA: Calcium channel blockers. In Stoelting RK (ed): Advances in Anesthesia, p 167. Chicago, Yearbook Medical Publishers, 1985

19. Gelmers HJ, Gorter K, DeWeedt CJ, et al: A controlled trial of nimodipine in acute ischemic stroke. N Engl J Med 318:203, 1988

20. Merin RG: Calcium channel blocking drugs and anesthetics: Is the drug interaction beneficial or detrimental? Anesthesiology 66:111, 1987

21. Merin RG, Chelly JE, Hysing ES, et al: Cardiovascular effects of and interaction between calcium blocking drugs and anesthetics in chronically instrumented dogs, IV: Chronically administered oral verapamil and halothane, enflurane and isoflurane. Anesthesiology 66:140, 1987

22. Slogoff S, Keats AS: Does chronic treatment with calcium entry blocking drugs reduce perioperative myocardial ischemia? Anesthesiology 68:676, 1988

23. Chung F, Huston PL, Cheng DCH, et al: Calcium channel blockade does not offer adequate protection from peri-operative myocardial ischemia. Anesthesiology 69:343, 1988

24. Singh DN, Opie LH, Marcus FI: Anti-arrhythmic agents. In Opie LH (ed): Drugs for the Heart , p 65. Orlando, Grune & Stratton 1984

25. Merin RG, Tonnesen AS: Cardiovascular effects of drug interactions between anesthetics and cardiovascular medications. In Altura B, Halevy S, (eds): Cardiovascular Actions of Anesthetics and Drugs Used in Anesthesia I, Basic Aspects, p 224. Zurich, S Karger, 1986

26. Gallagher JD, Lieverman RW, Meranze J, et al: Amiodarone-induced complications during coronary artery surgery. Anesthesiology 55:186, 1981

27. Smith TW: Digitalis: Mechanisms of action and clinical use. N Engl J Med 318:358, 1988
28. DiBianco R, Shabetai R, Kostu KW, et al: A comparison of oral milrinone, digoxin, and their combination in the treatment of patients with chronic heart failure. N Engl J Med 320:677, 1989
29. Jaski BE, Fifer MA, Wright RF, et al: Positive inotropic and vasodilator actions of milrinone in patients with severe congestive heart failure. J Clin Invest 75:643, 1985
30. Ludmer PL, Wright RF, Arnold JM, et al: Separation of the direct myocardial and vasodilator actions of milrinone administered by an intracoronary infusion technique. Circulation 73:130, 1986
31. Deutsch S, Dalen JE: Indications for prophylactic digitalization. Anesthesiology 30:648, 1969
32. Johnson LW, Dickstein RA, Fruehan CT, et al: Prophylactic digitalization for coronary artery bypass surgery. Circulation 53:819, 1976
33. Pinaud MLJ, Blanloeil YAG, Souron RJ: Preoperative prophylactic digitalization of patients with coronary artery disease: A randomized echocardiographic and hemodynamic study. Anesth Analg 62:865, 1983
34. Opie LH, Thadani U: Nitrates. In Opie LH (ed): Drugs for the Heart, p 23. Orlando, Grune & Stratton, 1985
35. Merin RG, Bastron RD: Diuretics. In Smith NT, Corbascio AN (ed): Drug Interactions in Anesthesia, 2nd ed. p 206. Philadelphia, Lea & Febiger, 1986
36. El-Ganzouri AR, Ivankovich AD, Braverman B, et al: Monoamine oxidase inhibitors: Should they be discontinued preoperatively? Anesth Analg 64:592, 1985
37. Wells DG, Bjorksten AR: Monoamine oxidase inhibitors revisited. Can J Anaesth 36:64, 1989
38. Stack CG, Rogers P, Linters PK: Monoamine oxidase inhibitors in anesthesia: A review. Br J Anaesth 60:222, 1988

Index

Page numbers in *italics* indicate illustrations; page numbers followed by (t) indicate tables.

A

Adrenergic receptors, 141–143
Alpha-adrenergic agonists, 147–148
Alpha-adrenergic antagonists, 148–149
Anesthesia
  antiarrhythmic drugs and, 155(t)
  in bronchoscopy, 133
  in thoracic surgery, noncardiac, 133–134
  in thoracotomy and lung resection, 133–134
  in upper abdominal surgery postoperative, 136–137
Angiography, radionuclide
  first pass, 30–31, *31*, 33(t)
  in mitral regurgitation evaluation, 66–67
Angiotensin-converting enzyme inhibitors, 149–150
Aortic regurgitation
  inotropy in, 61–62
  left ventricle volume overload in, 60–63, *61–62*
  pathophysiology of, 60–63, *61–62*
Aortic stenosis (AS), 105–107
  left ventricle pressure overload in, 67, *68*, 69, *70–72*, 71–72
  physiology of and risk for, 106(t)
  risk assessment of
    cardiac catheterization in, *74*, 75
    echocardiography in, 73, *74*
    perioperative, 58
    intravascular fluid therapy in, 73–74
    for valve replacement, 75–76
  valvulotomy in
    balloon, 76, 106

  surgical, 106–107
Arterial switch operation, 114
Atrioventricular canal defects, 104–105
  physiology of and risk for, 104(t)
AS. *See* Aortic stenosis
ASD. *See* Atrial septal defect
Atrial septal defect (ASD), 101

B

Balloon valvuloplasty
  in aortic stenosis, 76, 106
Beta-adrenergic agonists, 143
Beta-adrenergic antagonists
  pharmacokinetics of, 144(t), 144–145
  pharmacologic properties of, 144(t), 145
  preoperative considerations and, 146–147
  uses of, 146, 147, 155(t)
Blalock-Taussig shunt, 107
Bronchoscopy
  anesthesia in, 133
Bronchospirometry
  for split-function data, 128–129

C

CAD. *See* Coronary artery disease
Calcium channel-blockers
  clinical effects of, 151(t)
  comparison of, 153
  pharmacology of, 151–152
  preoperative considerations and, 153–154
  uses of, 152–153

Cardiac catheterization
  in aortic stenosis assessment, 74,
    75
  in congenital heart disease,
    95–96, 97, 98
  in ischemic heart disease,
    33–34, 34(t)
Cardiac mechanisms
  radionuclear evaluation of,
    30–33, 31, 33(t)
Cardiac output measurement, 35,
  36(t)
Cardiovascular medications
  angiotensin-converting enzyme
    inhibitors, 149–150
  anti-arrhythmic agents, 154–156,
    155(t)
  calcium channel-blockers,
    150–154, 151(t), 155(t)
  diuretics, 160–161, 161(t)
  inotropic agents, 156–159
  monoamine oxidase inhibitors,
    162–163
  sympathetic nervous system
    agonists and antagonists,
    141–149
    adrenergic receptor physiology
      and, 141–143
    alpha-adrenergic agonists,
      147–148
    alpha-adrenergic antagonists,
      148–149
    beta-adrenergic agonists, 143
    beta-adrenergic antagonists,
      143–147, 144(t)
    catecholamine-depleting
      agents, 149
  vasodilators, 159–160
Catecholamine-depleting drugs,
  149
CHD. *See* Congenital heart disease
Chest radiography
  in CHD, 93–94
  in ischemic heart disease, 8

Chronic obstructive pulmonary
  disease (COPD)
  in lung cancer, 125
  nonthoracic surgery and,
    134–135, 135
  pulmonary artery hypertension
    and, 130
Coarctation of the aorta, 108–109
  physiology of and risk for, 108(t)
Congenital heart disease (CHD)
  arterial switch operation in, 114
  atrial repair in, 113–114
  cardiac risk factors in, 98–99
    in corrected CHD, 99–101,
      100(t)
    in uncorrected CHD, 99, 99(t)
  congestive heart failure in,
    87–88
  dysrhythmias in, 88–89
  Fontan procedure in, 115–117,
    116(t)
  mitral valve replacement in, in
    children, 109–110, 110(t)
  obstruction to left heart outflow
    in, 89–90
  perioperative assessment
    methods in, 91(t)
    cardiac catheterization, 95–96,
      97, 98
    chest X-ray, 93–94
    echocardiography, 94–95
    history, 91–92
    laboratory tests, 93
    physical examination, 92–93
  pulmonary blood flow, 86–87
  specific lesions
    aortic stenosis, 105–107, 106(t)
    atrioventricular canal defects
      104(t), 104–105
    atrial septal defect, 101
    coarctation of the aorta, 108(t),
      108–109
    patent ductus arteriosus,
      101–102

systemic-to-pulmonary artery palliative shunts, 107(t), 107–108
ventricular septal defect, 102–104, 103(t)
tetralogy of Fallot, 110–111, 111(t)
corrected, 111–112
total anomalous pulmonary venous connection, 115, 115(t)
transposition of the great arteries, 112(t), 112–113
Congestive heart failure
in congenital heart disease, 87–88
in mitral regurgitation, 64–65, 64–65
COPD. *See* Chronic obstructive pulmonary disease (COPD)
Coronary angioplasty, 44
Coronary arteriography, 43–44
Coronary artery disease (CAD)
on chest radiography, 8
contrast echocardiography in, 19
on electrocardiograph, 6–7
on exercise stress test, 9, 13
on laboratory tests, 5
on physical examination, 4–5
ST-segment response in, 10, 11

D
Digitalis, 156–157, 158
Diuretics, 160–161, 161(t)
Dysrhythmias
in coronary heart disease, 88–89

E
Echocardiography
contrast, 19–22, *20*

Doppler, 18, 66
in aortic stenosis evaluation, 73
in congenital heart disease, 95
in mitral regurgitation evaluation, 66
M-mode, 14, *15*, 16
transesophageal two-dimensional, 16–17, *17*
two-dimensional, 16–17, *17*
Electrocardiography
in coronary artery disease, 6–7
in ischemic heart disease, 6–8
Exercise stress testing
angina and, 8–9, 12–13
coronary artery disease and, 9, 13
dysrhythmia detection via, 13–14
protocols for, *10*

F
Fontan procedure, 115–117, 116(t)

G
Gated blood-pool imaging, 31–32, 33(t)

H
Hemodynamic decompensation
in mitral regurgitation, 65
Hemodynamic measurements
of cardiac output, 35, 36(t)
of coronary sinus flow, 39–40
of oxygen consumption, 37
valve area calculation and, 38–39
of vascular resistance, 37–38
Hydralazine, 159–160

I

Inotropic drugs
  digitalis, 156–157, 158
  new agents, 157–158
  preoperative considerations and,
    158–159
Inotropy vs. systolic performance
  in valvular heart disease, 59–60,
    59–60
Ischemic heart disease
  cardiac catheterization in, 33–34,
    34(t)
  chest radiography in, 8
  coronary arteriography in,
    43–44
  echocardiography in, 14–22, *15,
    17, 20. See also* Contrast
    echocardiography
  electrocardiography in, 6–8
  exercise stress testing in, 8–9,
    10, 12–13
  hemodynamic measurements in,
    35, 36(t), 37–40
  laboratory tests in, 5–6, *6*
  left ventricular function in, as-
    sessment of, 4
  magnetic resonance imaging and
    spectroscopy in, 44–45
  nuclear imaging in, 22–24, *25,
    26–30, 27–28,* 28(t)
  physical examination in, 4–5
  preoperative syndromes in,
    2–4
  radionuclear evaluation in, of
    cardiac mechanisms, 30–33,
    31, 33(t)
  ST-segment response and,
    9–12
  ventriculography in, 40–42,
    41

J

Jatene repair, 114

L

Lateral position test
  for split-function data, 129–130
Left ventricle
  in aortic stenosis
    pressure overload of, 67, *68,
      69, 70–72, 71–72*
  in aortic regurgitation,
    volume overload of, 60–63,
      61–62
  in mitral stenosis
    volume underload in, 76–81
Lung(s). *See also entries beginning
    with* Pulmonary
  split-function studies of,
    128–130
Lung cancer
  chronic obstructive pulmonary
    disease and, 125
  thoracotomy and resection in,
    125–134
Lung scanning, perfusion, 129

M

Magnetic resonance imaging,
  44–45
Minoxidil, 159–160
Mitral regurgitation
  myocardial depression in, 63, *64,*
    65
  pressure-volume in, 63, *64*
  risk assessment of
    for noncardiac surgery 64–65
    Doppler echocardiography
      and, 66
    radionuclide angiography in,
      66–67
    sequential pacing and, 66
Mitral stenosis (MS)
  pathophysiology of, 76–78
  perioperative risk of, 58
  pulmonary hypertension in,
    77–78

risk assessment of
pulmonary function test in,
78–79
for prosthetic valve replacement, 79–80
Mitral valve replacement
in children, 109–110, 110(t)
prosthetic, 79–80
M-mode echocardiography, 14, *15*,
16
Monoamine oxidase inhibitors,
162–163
MS. *See* Mitral stenosis
Myocardial infarction, preexisting,
3–4
Myocardial ischemia, silent, 3–4
Myocardium
in valvular heart disease
systolic performance vs.
inotropy in, 59–60, *60*
wall motion evaluation of,
19–21, *20*

Positron-emission tomography, cardiac, 23
Potts shunt, 108
Pulmonary artery hypertension,
130–131
Pulmonary artery pressure monitoring
in mitral regurgitation
preoperative, 66
Pulmonary blood flow
in congenital heart disease,
86–87
Pulmonary function
criteria and risk in, 127–128, *128*
exercise studies of, 131–132
in mitral stenosis, 78–79
postsectional, 134
spirometric studies of, 126–129,
127
split-function studies of,
128–130
vascular catheterization studies
of, 130–131

N
Nuclear imaging, 22–23
in angiography, first pass,
30–31, *31*, 33(t)
cold spot, 26–27, *27*, 28(t)
gated blood-pool study, 31–32,
33(t)
hot spot, with technetium-99m,
24, *25*, 26, 28(t)
thallium-201 perfusion and,
27–28, *29*

P
Patent ductus arteriosus, 101–102
Perfusion lung scanning, 129
Pneumonectomy, vascular catheter-
ization studies of, postopera-
tive, 130–131

R
Radionuclide angiography
in mitral regurgitation, 66–67
Radiospirometry
for split-function data, 129

S
Shunts
systemic-to-pulmonary-artery,
107–108
Blalock-Taussig, 107
physiology of and risk for,
107(t)
Potts, 108
Waterston, 108
Spirometry
bronchospirometry, 128–129

Spirometry (*continued*)
   in pulmonary function evalua-
      tion, baseline, 126–128, *128*
   radiospirometry, 129
Surgery
   nonthoracic
      chronic obstructive pulmonary
         disease and, 134–135, *135*
      postoperative anesthetic man-
         agement in, 136–137
      risk reduction in, 136
      ventilatory defect in, 135
   thoracic, 125–134
Systolic performance vs. inotropy
   in valvular heart disease, 59–60,
      59–60

T

Technetium-99m pyrophosphatase,
   in nuclear imaging, 24, *25*,
   26, 28(t)
Tetralogy of Fallot, 110–111, 111(t)
   corrected, 111–112
Thallium-201 imaging, 26–27, *27*
Thiazide diuretics, 160–161, 161(t)
Thoracic surgery, noncardiac. *See*
   Surgery, nonthoracic; Thoracotomy and lung resection
Thoracotomy and lung resection
   anesthesia in, 133–134
   patient evaluation for, 125–126,
      126(t)
   pulmonary function testing and,
      126–133, *127*, 128(t), *132*
Thrombolysis, intracoronary,
   44–45
Total anomalous pulmonary
   venous connection, 115,
   115(t)
Transposition of the great arteries,
   112–113

physiology of and risk factors
   for, 112(t)

V

Valve area calculation, 39–40
Valvular heart disease (VHD)
   aortic and mitral regurgitation in,
      60–63, *61–62*
   aortic stenosis in, 67, *68*, 69,
      70–72, 71–76, *74*
   mitral regurgitation in, 63, *64*,
      65–67
   mitral stenosis in, 76–80
   myocardium in
      systolic performance vs.
         inotropy, 59–60, *59–60*
   perioperative risk in, 57–59
Valvulotomy
   balloon, 76, 106
   surgical, 106–107
Vascular resistance measurement,
   37–38
Vasodilators, direct, 159–160
Ventricular function
   contrast echocardiographic
      assessment of, 21–22
Ventricular septal defect (VSD),
   102–104
   physiology of and risk for, 103(t)
Ventriculography
   in ischemic heart disease,
      40–42, *41*
VHD. *See* Valvular heart disease
VSD. *See* Ventricular septal defect

W

Waterston shunt, 108

ISBN 0-397-51089-6

90000

9 780397 510894